"This lovely book is, in its entirety, a _____ love, middle-aged love, and love that endures through the profound changes of Alzheimer's and on into the loneliness and mystery of death. It has two authors, two poets, Diana Saltoon, and her late husband Robert Briggs. In these pages Robert is quite alive, even as his own memory—but not his sense of humor—fades. Although it is quite interesting to read this touching memoir and to learn about the Beat generation from one who lived it, it is their Zen practice that shines through, and the book's unexpected effect is a warming, spreading radiance in the reader's heart."

—Jan Chozen Bays, MD, and co-abbot of Great Vow Zen Monastery in Clatskanie, Oregon, is also a pediatrician who specializes in child abuse and is author of several books including *Mindful Eating: A Guide to Rediscovering a Healthy and Joyful Relationship with Food* and *How to Train a Wild Elephant: And Other Adventures in Mindfulness.*

"The authors Diana Saltoon and the late Robert Briggs write a love story through the eyes of poetry, Zen, and the relief from suffering, which is love. Deep bows to this blessed wisdom and compassion and to the authors."

—Larry Christensen, PhD, is the Head Teacher at The Zen Center of Portland and a clinical psychologist in Portland, OR.

"From the overlapping poetry and prose of Robert and Diana, we gain insight into how the interests they shared throughout their long marriage—prose, poetry, jazz, politics, Japanese tea ceremony, existentialism, and Zen—sustain them. They reach a place where fragments of language and the gestures of everyday life bring them to an understanding of each other that transcends words."

—Clayton Morgareidge, Professor Emeritus, Lewis and Clark College, author of *Demystifying Demons: Rethinking Who and What We Are.*

To: Eileen

Thanks for all you do! I wanted to share this book with you.... its special to me.

Best-

Angus

6/8/16

Wife, Just Let Go

WIFE, JUST LET GO

Zen, Alzheimer's, and Love

* * *

Robert Briggs & Diana Saltoon

ROBERT BRIGGS ASSOCIATES
Portland, Oregon

Published by Robert Briggs Associates
Copyright © 2017 by Diana Saltoon

Wife, Just Let Go: Zen, Alzheimer's, and Love
a duo-memoir by Robert Briggs & Diana Saltoon
(1. Zen. 2. Alzheimer's Disease. 3. Care-giving. 4. Love. 5. Poetry.
6. Beat Generation. 7. Jazz.)

Designed by Mark Ong, Side By Side Studios, San Francisco, CA

Cover photo by Christine Toth, Portland, OR

ISBN: 978-0-931191-20-6

For Robert

& Hillary

Contents

Face to Face

DIANA

You don't really know who
you truly are.
You see an aging face and body
hear a name or words describing "me."
The self with a given name
changes with circumstances
fashioned out of conditions
in time only fleeting.

Dearest, if you want to know
the incredible being you are
enter within the deep silence
in endless space before a sound
or ripple of thought or word.
Here, in unmeasured love,
we may embrace
face—to original face.

D.S.

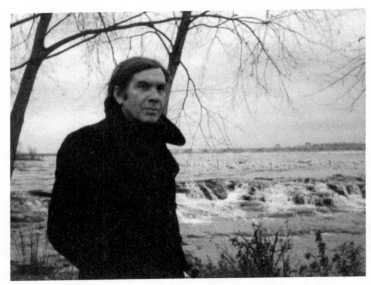

Robert at Niagara Falls, NY, 1979, during a visit to Mad Bear, an American
Indian medicine man of the Bear Clan of the Tuscarora Nation.

Preface

DIANA

This book began with a promise I made to my husband, Robert Briggs, that I would somehow find a way to see his last work in print, written after he received a diagnosis of Alzheimer's. Concerned by the doctor's statement of his condition, he returned to his makeshift desk at his daughter's home and continued to write. He had turned eighty-three and writing was something that still moved and inspired him beyond all other activities. And, as before, he felt the crucial need to rewrite or edit what he wrote. Even as the disease progressed, he was always holding a pen or pencil or a small bottle of whiteout to blot out words he thought no longer useful for a particular phrase or sentence. To the very end of his life, he held a pen and scrap of paper to jot down notes and thoughts. This instinct to refine the written page never left him.

As his wife, companion, and creative partner, I accompanied Robert on this journey as best I could, as I had before his diagnosis. As his primary care-person, experiencing, day-by-day, the wrenching loss of my loved one's brain, I turned to poetry for relief and expression. As I began to compile his essays, I realized that there was more to his work—a lifetime of memories and a story of love, and so began this dual memoir of a life together that ended in a journey of Alzheimer's. The project grounded me as later, oceans of grief overwhelmed the first weeks and months after he died.

Towards the end of Robert's Alzheimer's journey, old and dear friends welcomed us back to Portland, and embraced us with their love and support. It is for them, and Robert, and for all others with loved ones struggling with this disease, that I'm inspired to join Robert in this book.

Robert's reflections do not mention his disease, although it haunts every word and line of his work. Things became more difficult after he turned eighty-five, and though he continued to write, he struggled to share the poignant and joyous *now* of each moment he met with his heart rather than his head. For Robert, love came to rule the day. Much of what he shares is about aging, as well as what he calls "vital aging," the latter having more to do with the "qi or chi" of one's inner energy, its weakness or strength. In Robert's case, he found meditation a sure way to enhance his own "qi," something that translated into his belief in the "power of aging."

1

For Robert at Eighty-Three

DIANA

Your Birthday always
a day to celebrate
remember the love
the decades together.

Now turning eighty-three
young as ever
you smile swinging
on a park swing.

Age is intolerant
of those who organize
hours, days, weeks
putting life on shelves
like books unread
but oh, they decorate.
You've never left
a book unturned
a question unexplored.

This birthday
precious and tender
this knowing you
being with you
years of grace and
sweet appreciation.

Looking back with wonder
what circumstances—
conditions—synced
that day we met
and recognized
our strange cousin-try.
What planets—sun
moon—stars—ordained
this flow of oneness
not undisturbed
to carry us here—now
as we are.

D.S.

2

On My Eighty-Third Birthday, June, 2012

ROBERT, 2012, NEW YORK

After so many birthdays I can hardly begin to remember where I might have started from. Sometimes I strain to wonder, but that never changes anything until I realize what remembered birthdays might lead to—if each were patiently recalled and, studied in some kind of order, might just allow me to create an unusual history of my life.

No one really knows where they started from, and few know why. Yet that is no reason to change anything. After a while, change becomes a wondrous quest.

I soon learned there is much to do, but little need to hurry. Only to walk on by whatever bothers me because I realize there is always a way to begin, because any cool need contains precious ideas.

So now, at eighty-three, I realize I have an unusual opportunity to sanely rise every morning and enjoy the sun or the rain. Yet I still have a loving need to continue to look for ideas or thoughts that might turn into an inspiration—

whether it is a question or a need to wonder why life can be so amazing.

At eighty-three, there is no need to avoid anything. If the sky is incredible, it should be used to see more than is sometimes seen, or more than is expected—such as when friends call just to ask "Hey! What's new?"

There is no reason not to believe that your life will be wise. All that's needed is faith in whatever comes, to remind you that there are even ways to solve the problems of friends, because at eighty-three, there are continuous reasons to believe that a good life can resolve anything. By using imagination and intuition you can know more than is known— in order to expand your consciousness. And there are ways to discover truth and love by having faith in silence and the many different ways that life goes on, in spite of old age and a growing loss of memory.

Often, I gaze out of windows and over streets and lawns and other familiar spaces—just to remember where I came from and where to go whenever I need to remember who I am. I do this in order to shed light on wherever I am.

I was born in Omaha, Nebraska, just before the crash of 1929. By the time I was in high school, my family moved to New Jersey where I attended Dwight Morrow High School and the Englewood School for Boys.

From there I went down south to Auburn University where I played in ruthless games of football—until I heard about French existentialism which redefined choice and action for me in a world I was continuously trying to understand.

I left Auburn to study and play football at the University of Chattanooga for two semesters. Then I joined my family back in New Jersey where—one day—the radio announced that an airplane had hit the top of the Empire State Building! I excitedly took a bus into New York City where I looked up with hundreds of others to see that an American bomber had hit the top of the Empire State Building! The sight was astonishing. But when the police cordoned off the area, I was forced to go home, where I could not stop talking about what I had seen.

3

An Unanticipated Circus

ROBERT, 2012, NEW YORK

Life in America is often like an unanticipated circus. You never know exactly what it will be like until you experience it.

I have always had wonderful expectations, many of which were realized. Yet, at eighty-three, I wait for more—knowing what to do because I know now what *not* to do. Over the years I have learned how to acknowledge and balance both weakness and strength in the many unexpected turns of life.

Moreover, in the reality of modern America, it is necessary to be able to deal with sudden change. This, however, is demanding because one has to get out of one's comfort zone to accept any true change.

I often wonder if at times my life is like a deserted circus. Once ended, it will leave only fond memories of what I enjoyed—the thrill of the wonderful booming music; the screech of elephants; the roar of magnificent tigers; and the incredible high-wire flying acrobats who dive and lock hands with each other. There is great beauty to the graceful swing of these acrobats and how change is made by the high flyers who fall and grip one another in mid-air in time to make a fear-struck audience suddenly stand and burst into explosive screams that incite the orchestra into rounds of fantastic music.

Unfortunately, this kind of circus seems to be a thing of the past. At eighty-three, my joyful circus is an after-glow of memories that seem to return whenever I remember marvelous times in my life.

DIANA

In 2012, Robert's "joyful circus" of memories was slipping away. To recapture "those marvelous times," I hoped to be a kind of memory bank for him, gifting memories he's lost, cherished moments, and other experiences that brought special turns in our life together. I encouraged reminisces of his early life and, as much as I could, reminded him of events written in his memoir of the 1950s, his passionate love of poetry, and the root of that love, beginning in a memory of his father.

4

My First Interest in Poetry

ROBERT, 2012, NEW YORK

I began to read poetry while in high school. My father so liked my interest in poetry that we often shared poems and poets together. I now realize this gave me something to be serious about—something that always lasted, for he gave a piece of his heart whenever he read a poem. I treasured this memory in later years.

I wrote more poetry but showed it to few, because those who said they loved poetry seemed to know so much more about it than I did that I hesitated joining them.

5

Some Favorite Poems

ROBERT, 2012, NEW YORK

The following lines of W.H. Auden describe in part
some of the magic, mystery, and allure of his work:

> For poetry makes nothing happen: it survives
> in the valley of its making where executives
> would never want to tamper, flows on south
> from ranches of isolation and the busy griefs,
> raw towns that we believe and die in;

Another poem that has always haunted me is Thomas
Hardy's "Lizbie Browne," especially these lines:

> Dear Lizbie Browne—
> Where are you now?
> In sun, in rain?—
> Or is your brow
> Past joy, past pain? . . .

> Dear Lizbie Browne,
> I should have thought,
> "Girls ripen fast,"
> And coaxed and caught
> You ere you passed,
> Dear Lizbie Browne! . . .

But, Lizbie Browne,
I let you slip;

So, Lizbie Browne,
When on a day
Men speak of me
As not, you'll say,
"And who was he?"—
Yes, Lizbie Browne!"

... Sweet Lizbie Brown.
Oh, yes—Lizbie Brown.

DIANA

Why did that particular poem of Thomas Hardy's *Lizbie Browne* interest Robert? A romantic at heart, Robert loved Hardy's descriptions of a love that never was but could have been.

In New York, reflecting on his early life, his mind steadily slipping from him, *Lizbie Browne* stayed an inspiration along with T.S. Eliot's, *The Love Song of J. Alfred Prufrock.* He was drawn to Prufrock's struggle to make a genuine contact with love, to find meaning in the ruins of a modern city, his anxieties around time. These were themes that touched Robert and stayed with him—love, a decline of modern life about him, the concern with time and memory.

As Eliot says in Prufrock:

> ... I am no prophet — and here's no great matter;
> I have seen the moment of my greatness flicker,
> And I have seen the eternal Footman hold my coat, and
>   snicker,
> And in short, I was afraid. ...

Robert continued to be drawn to Eliot and how words could portray the innermost feelings of a writer through a fictionalized character yet keep private the "within" of the writer himself.

In New York, the Alzheimer's disease draws Robert even more deeply into this "private within."

Influenced by Eliot, Robert wrote this poem in his younger days back in San Francisco:

A FEW LINES OFF TOM ELIOT,
RECENTLY OF ST. LOUIS
WOOD TUESDAY

Because I don't intend to burn again!
Because I don't intend
I am willing to try anything
Because I don't intend to forget.

Because I'm not sure time isn't overrated
and real estate wouldn't be smarter after all.
I think my Lord is kidding.

Because I don't intend to burn again
consequently I am peeved,
having to blame somebody for the joke.

I pray to God to quit kidding
and pray I may remember
when this charade was first taken seriously,
first incorporated.

Smile now and at the hour of our rebirth.
Smile now and at the hour of rebirth.

R.B.

A strange poem. What did it have to do with Eliot? However, I could never get Robert to explain that one to me or some of his earlier poems which he read at the San Francisco Jazz Cellar back in the 1950s. He called them three short "jazz regrets" in his book: *Ruined Time: The 1950s and the Beat*:

> After all the life
> about me, with me,
> I want to go back to
> the womb—I do!
> Any old womb will do.
> I must have left something behind.
>
> *
>
> Oh! I don't care
> who He is
> if he drops
> that cross again he's
> out of the parade!
> And no way!
> No way!
> Do those relatives
> get any nails!
>
> *
>
> Lay your myopic head
> on my laundry bag, beloved!
> It'll be months
> before
> the Red Cross gets here.
>
> R.B.

I often quoted his book to him, or placed it near where he could easily pick it up, leaf through its pages picking out thoughts and recollections from them. Robert's prose in 2012, when he turned eighty-three, was certainly simpler, briefer. Though his hands would tremble, he was still able to sign his name on a form or a check. Robert continued writing through 2012, reflecting about the time he left college.

6

Just Out of College

ROBERT, 2012, NEW YORK

In early 1950, out of college, I was drafted into the army and sent to Fort Bliss, Texas, for training where I emerged a Second Lieutenant and—six months later—was sent to war in Korea. Fortunately, the Korean War suddenly ended and I was shipped back to the States and released from military duty. This allowed me to enter Columbia University on the G.I. Bill, where I studied creative writing with a keen professor who taught me how to write—something I had wanted to do since I was very young. At that point in life, I loved to write. Yet, as a beginner, I seldom liked much of what I wrote, as it often felt mundane until I was drawn back into French existentialism. During the 1950s, this new school of thought offered new ways to deepen my thinking and widen my interests. It also led to writers I had previously ignored. This made me realize that, since I so badly wanted to write, I needed to be more serious about it. I soon found that even good writing needed to be rewritten several times in order to create something meaningful.

In the 1950s French existentialism was not only a unique way of thinking but offered alternatives to ordinary life, which made existentialism a worldwide sensation. Outside of France, the ideals of existentialism were easily adapted to many cultures and languages. The need to live a larger life—a core ideal of existentialism—is universally understood. I recognized it was something I needed to do, so I started to do so.

This enhanced my writing and made me realize other ways of opening my heart as well as my mind. It seemed to lead into what became an imaginary but dimly anticipated circus—a circus before the activity begins—a time when I met all kinds of same-minded people looking for ways to live larger lives that were more honest and meaningful. This created in me a need to step out into a challenging, information-oriented world in order to find answers.

DIANA

Once in a while, an old memory would come up and Robert would smile. "So," I'd probe a bit, "what's on your mind?" One day he brought up war.

"It's my Uncle Leo," he said, "he always used to make me laugh—but I remember when he returned from his stint as a seaman in World War II, he didn't joke as much and didn't stay in Omaha. He went to Los Angeles where he felt money could be made. Like so many others, he was sick of war."

"Remember the poem of Randall Jarrell you loved about the war?" I asked.

He shook his head. I found the page in *Ruined Time* where he quoted Jarrell and asked him to read it:

> In bombers named for girls, we burned
> the cities we had learned about in school
> till our lives wore out; our bodies lay among
> the people we had killed and never seen.
> When we lasted long enough they gave us medals;
> when we died they said, "Our casualties were low."

I never tired hearing him read. His voice was still as cadent as ever, though not as strong. He mentioned the atomic bomb "Little Boy," dropped on Hiroshima in 1945 by the U.S. government "killing all those people." He shook his head. "But that wasn't enough so they dropped another one, 'Fat Man'—another atomic horror that was to end all wars." ("Little Boy" was the codename for the atomic bomb dropped on the Japanese city of Hiroshima on August 6, 1945, during World War II, and "Fat Man" the code for the atomic bomb detonated over the Japanese city of Nagasaki by the U.S. on August 9, 1945.)

At his improvised desk, slightly hunched in his chair facing his old computer, he wrote of his own experience with that horror of all arsenals—the Atom Bomb.

7

My Own Atom Bomb

ROBERT, 2005, OREGON,

REVISED IN 2012, NEW YORK

More than eight years after atomic bombs were dropped on Hiroshima and Nagasaki and ended WW2 in 1945, the US, spurred by a fear of communism, continued to test its arsenal of atomic bombs at sites in the Pacific Ocean and the Nevada Desert.

Even knowing the devastating results of those bombs dropped in Japan, it still seemed never enough. Not enough to realize that nuclear weapons eclipsed any holocaust and topped the score of inhumanity. No. More proof was needed and more statistics had to be found.

So! Back in 1953, as an army officer in Ft. Belvoir, Virginia, I was ordered with my platoon to fly out to Nevada and observe and experience firsthand an atomic explosion up close. An experience I was assured would let me live to fight another day. I was one of many second lieutenants sent out by the government on a "Secret Mission" to test the effects of an Atom Bomb blast on human beings as well as animals and equipment.

The night before it happened, I wandered around Las Vegas, in and out of the noisy din of bright casinos that spun all kinds of scenes in my head, until I caught a cab at midnight and went back to BOQ (Bachelor Officer Quarters). After a short sleep, I woke up, put on a pair of combat boots, picked up a steel helmet and reported before 0-300 hours to a nearby staging area which was over a low hill. As I got to the top, I heard the growl of many idling engines and looked down on a monstrous circle of flood lights under which stretched endless lines of two-and-a-half-ton trucks full of GIs who must have been on those rigs for ten or more hours. On my way down the hill, the scene seemed Hollywood-ish until I got there and was approached by a young Atomic Energy messenger who sped up in a jeep and handed me a small film badge to pin on my top pocket. This badge, which I would have to turn in following the test, was not for identification purposes but would measure radiation. It came with an info sheet that again warned me that the exercise was TOP SECRET and, because of possible contamination, outer garments might have to be discarded. Might? But by then it was too late to ask because everything seemed as meaningless as the vast Nevada sprawl, because long lines of trucks began to creep past the flood-lit gathering and slow down to allow the convoy to pass over to the flat. After my truck arrived, that flat seemed like an endless curve of purple moonscape, an unbelievable sight especially after I got out. Frenchman Flat was scarred by a sea of shallow slit trenches that circled a huge, black, flood-lit, Eiffel-like tower that was topped by an enormous box from which thick bunches of fat and thin cables and spiral wires were plugged into huge space crates. As I gazed around, the sharp voice of a captain behind me snapped and told me to entrench my men and after the blast lead them to the tower.

Once that captain left, a sergeant showed me how to cover my "holes"—to use my thumbs to shut my ears, press my fingers over my eye-lids and nostrils and squeeze my lips closed, which I later found out was a two-handed face clamp left over from World War One. Something you did then when there was no time to put on a gas mask.

So, no matter what time it was, I closed all of my holes just as an unseen loud speaker began an exaggerated final countdown, during which I wormed my knees and wriggled both elbows deeper into the ground of a shallow four-foot slit trench until I heard the final "two-ah, one-ah," and then "zee-row"! After which—a sudden split of a second later—an immense blast of rushed and roaring hot needles and slick silver lights shot through my finger-pressed eyelids and created a hissing absence of air. This was followed by a huge typhoon "woosh" of combustion that lifted and twisted and dipped the trench I was in—until I was looking down on the men below me then up at helmets

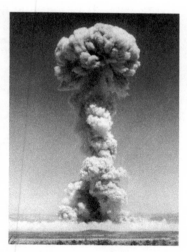

Atomic Bomb explosion, 1951 (Location NTS, Areas 1-4, 6-10, Yucca Flat, NV). Photo rendered by Chel White, Portland, OR

above me as the trench continued to quiver and shake and dip! As a fierce mass of hell-propelled filth sped so fast over my head that it seemed as if the earth was whizzing around the universe. Until moments or minutes later after I let go of my last hole I was slowly able to stand up.

It seemed as if the sun had pushed heaven down in order to illuminate a huge circle of overhead dust under which I was able to wobble up and out of the trench. Ground Zero turned out to be nothing—nothing but a huge smooth empty circle of earth about fifty yards away where the metal shell of a two-and-a-half-ton truck was smoking upside down. It was as if the world went with it.

That was an atom bomb—a monstrous blast of light and heat and might that forever reoriented my mind and refined my imagination until thirty or forty hours later when I was flying back to DC in another rattling C-47, I feared my brain had been scorched or celestially swept away by some force I couldn't get away from. From some uncertain reverberation, some rip of hellish fear that some razor shade of me would always be marooned out on Frenchman Flat.

DIANA

Was Robert's Alzheimer's disease some lingering malignant outcome of that mushroom cloud he observed above his head at Frenchman Flat? The mystery of the disease is such that there is no way to know how and from where it comes.

The degree of fallout Robert experienced was never revealed to him. The badge, if it measured anything, was taken from him immediately after the test. Also, his badge had no ID on it, so it precluded any inquiry about the contamination experienced. Speculation continues regarding many of the diseases—leukemia; lymphoma; thyroid; breast and bone cancers; gastrointestinal tract cancers; brain tumors—that may have developed from the fallout of Nevada mushroom clouds. Robert wondered how those in his platoon out at Frenchman Flat survived after that experience. He had felt it intensely—it seared into his flesh. He hated any kind of arsenal and never desired or owned a firearm.

When anyone asks Robert why he escaped those cancers, he replies, "Because I covered my holes."

He understood my childhood fear of men in military uniforms—something inherited from World War II when, as an infant in Singapore, my family and I were interned during the Japanese occupation. That fear would revisit me sometimes at the sight of an armed policeman approaching my car or on the street. Robert would then place an arm about me or hold my hand tighter. I'd feel secure then, protected by his love and tenderness. Later, much later, as he grew weaker, I still felt that security every time he held my hand.

8

A Crack in the Bowl

DIANA

A CRACK IN THE BOWL

We were young when we married
now growing old together
we face our vow
of "sickness and health."

No one warned
of brain decline, dementia
or worse the name—
Alzheimer.

Love that bonds cannot ignore
the slow loss of the other.
Grieving begins
with no end
freedom no longer
an option or desire.

Pain unseen
lifted in a moment's ease

returns again twice-fold
to tease
Patience,
with a scream inside:
anything but this!

D.S.

In November of 2011, just before Robert's diagnosis, we left our dear friends of twenty years in Oregon to start a life in New York with Robert's daughter and son-in-law. Many circumstances led to this big decision and transition. The major reason was a need for Robert to reconnect with his family, especially his daughter, Hillary. Robert's only sister, Betty Jo, was still alive in 2011 though ailing. She lived in New Jersey where her son and his wife and family also lived. Robert wished to renew what had been a long distance relationship with them. Other reasons were financial, as we found ourselves at ages eighty-two and seventy-one forced to sell our house on a short sale (part of the many effected by the 2008 Wall Street financial debacle) and dwindling savings. Thinking to pool our resources and recoup through writing and sales of our published books and CDs, we settled in a home with Hillary and her husband.

Used to having my own home since Robert and I met thirty-five years ago, I was willing to go along until we could establish our own place nearby. These hopes came crashing down a few months after our arrival, when Robert suffered a bad fall landing on his head and chest. He was already having a memory issue (more evident to his daughter than us). It was then that Robert was connected to the Veterans Administration Hospital in the Bronx where he was thoroughly checked and an MRI performed on his brain.

Robert knew he was having memory issues but excused it as part of aging. After all, he felt that, at eighty-two going on eighty-three, he was entitled to some dementia. Even after his doctor blatantly mentioned Alzheimer's, both of us dismissed the diagnosis. In particular, I had great difficulty accepting it as Robert was still able to write and, when needed, perform one of his many jazz and poetry reads begun in Portland, Oregon, with a jazz trio. We hoped to continue those reads in New York and felt rather indignant about the diagnosis. It could not be! All kinds of thoughts assailed me. These were supposed to be our "golden years"—why this? Why now? Why us?

Robert's wise daughter, however, who had recently lost her grandmother (on her mother's side) to the disease, knew

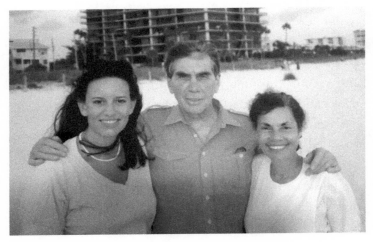

Hillary Briggs, Robert, and Diana in St. Petersburg, FL, 1989.
Photo by Will McGowan

better. She immediately set about researching all the information and assistance in New York. Through her amazing efforts we were able to cope for the next year or two following the Alzheimer's diagnosis, and Robert benefited from a clinical study offered at the VA Hospital through the Mt. Sinai School of Medicine in Manhattan.

During this time, Robert continued to write. It seemed all he could do to hang on to some stability, some inner core. He turned more to meditation and looked forward to receiving the bowl of whisked green tea I made, something I'd often prepare for him when we were in Oregon, where I taught the Japanese Way of Tea.

Robert's reflections written during those three years in New York are musings of stories past and present, an album of words. They are also testament of a brave heart and mind as it joins others on the path of Alzheimer's, seeking to live with purpose and human dignity even as the dark labyrinth of dementia slowly robs the mind.

9

On Dealing with Women

ROBERT, 2013, NEW YORK

Often, as I look back over the years, I think about the various fine women I've known. In the beginning, my mother and my sister were always "there for me" and were always honest about what I needed to hear, whether I liked it or not. As I grew up, much of it was not welcomed. Yet, after a while, I found that I valued their advice, realizing the wisdom of it. My only reservation was that it was usually advice that seemed to rob me of what I wanted to do—when what I had intended to do was hardly wise and, in the long run, a bit dumb.

Nevertheless, by the end of any week, I was asking for more advice because more was needed. I was smart enough to know where serious and experienced advice was to be found. It was with the two brightest women that I knew at that time.

Growing older I easily realized that I should know when and where I was—and where I shouldn't be. This allowed me to know about women and to often call or write my mother or my sister.

I learned how smart, loving, creative, helpful, generous, and stylish women are in their own unique and wonderful ways. Therefore, I knew to treat women with the respect they deserved.

I once had the pleasure of meeting a woman who impressed me so much that the experience of her presence still remains.

10

The Night I Met Eleanor Roosevelt

ROBERT, 2013, NEW YORK

I was working then at Newark Airport for Eastern Airlines. Newark in 1954 was a bustling international airport owned by the city of Newark and operated by the Port Authority of New York and New Jersey. Newark Airport was the first major airport in the United States. Eastern Airlines was quite popular then, and we were kept busy from morning to night by all kinds of travelers impatient to get to their various destinations.

Before I began work at Eastern, I tried my hand at selling cars in the shiny showroom of a dealership in New Jersey where I was hired to sell the latest Mercury Monterey sedan that had been secretly marked up an additional five hundred dollars over the dealer's top profit price and was then discounted to wow serious buyers into thinking it was a steal of a deal. That bit of wheeling and dealing created such a heartless drag in my head that after a week I left the dealership. After that stint I was happy to get a spot at the ticket counter at Newark Airport.

So, uniformed in Eastern's sky-blue shirt and dark blue trousers, I bobbed and weaved behind a high check-in counter that every morning and afternoon held at bay a bubbling rush of humble and haughty travelers hurrying to get off the ground. Sometimes dumbfounded by what they said and did to one another before scurrying off to board flights, I made mental notes as I wrote ticket after ticket and looped bag tags on mounds of luggage.

I was on a midnight shift the night I met Eleanor Roosevelt. She was and still is one of my favorite First Ladies of the White House. She was unusually outspoken, a powerhouse of a woman, a diplomat, activist and humanitarian, working on children's causes and women's rights, especially those of women correspondents and the League of Women Voters. She accepted countless national and international speaking and writing engagements. Later, she devoted herself to the work of the United Nations and traveled all over the world. Unpretentious and authentic, she was easily recognizable by the average American who found a champion in her. Wherever she went, her elegance and kindness stood out. You could not help but respect and admire her honesty and integrity.

As her flight approached the Eastern terminal, I got a call to meet a VIP arriving on the last plane from Washington, D.C. That VIP was of course, Eleanor Roosevelt. Shaking with awe and excitement, I hurried down the concourse to meet her flight. By the gate and above the concourse were several men in dark suits stationed discretely. I presumed they were Secret Service Agents assigned to her safety. The plane cruised in on time and had few passengers at that late hour. They were held back onboard so that she'd be the first to disembark. With excitement and some trepidation, hoping I'd not say or do the wrong thing, I waited for the door to open. I need not have worried. She came down the stairs and tired as she might have been, she gave me a big smile as I welcomed her. Her blue eyes were clear and direct as she looked at me and said, "thank you, young man, for meeting me." I gave her my arm and offered to carry her bag, but she insisted on carrying it herself and saying, "It keeps me fit, you see."

She wore a dark suit and sensible shoes and was tall and impressive, with graying hair neatly piled on top of her head in a bun. She took my arm as I escorted her out of the terminal into one of two waiting cars. The driver from the first car took her bag and placed it into the car. Before she got in, she turned to me, thanked me again, and gave me a warm handshake.

The Secret Service men got into the other car. As both cars sped away, I could still feel the warmth of that handshake. It had been more than an honor to have met her flight. It was a privilege I have never forgotten.

11

How Valued Still

DIANA

How valued still
the hours
as you move in
and out
within a dream that
brings us together
and moves us apart
with forgotten words
lost thoughts.

D.S.

Sometimes illness makes a person seem partial but they remain whole—no matter what. There are so many hidden treasures within a person to be discovered.

With Robert I learned patience, forgiveness and placing a great faith in love. Throughout his illness he never lost tenderness. Some of the books written about Alzheimer's can be depressing; I found few that addressed a care-person's hidden emotional grief and loss. Dealing with a loved one's daily needs is a journey often tested. It demands that we remain keenly aware of our personal emotional reactions at all times because those suffering from Alzheimer's have heightened sensitivity to emotional responses. An angry or irritated response from a care-person affects their condition adversely.

We had done so much together and now Alzheimer's was robbing us of life. Was I remiss in my own responses? Did I, as his care-person, scream against the day—the hour—the night?

"I can't take this anymore!" I'd yell in the privacy of the bathroom, letting the hot shower run, holding my head, and then scrubbing my face as if to wash it all away.

Yes, there were overpowering moments. Fear, anxiety, and despair engulfed me at times, especially when our economics became a pressing concern. It triggered forgetfulness of Robert's own anxieties. Feeling angry, confined, at times even caged because of the circumstances of Robert's disease, I'd lash out mindlessly with impatience and resentment over the loss of freedom to engage in my own activities. Though hurt, Robert was seldom reactive to my outbursts. A natural equanimity guided him throughout the years of his disease; but when things got heated or too frustrating, he'd stutter, grope for words, or, conversely, hold me tight, to reconnect to a softer part of me.

A few rare times, exasperated and confused, he'd physically shake me until I'd calm down. This made him sad, however. When the sadness got deep, there'd be tears in his eyes. Seeing him cry devastated me and I would turn against myself for hurting him. With deep regret, I'd put my head on his knees and beg his forgiveness. He'd answer, "no, no need to ask forgiveness."

Fortunately my spiritual training held up a mirror into my own separation and desires that created the very suffering I was trying to escape. It reminded me that our decades of tandem life, and support of caring family and friends were a blessing.

What helped, too, when an intense emotion threatened to disrupt, was to remember to breathe—to pause and take a deep breath before reacting. This practice became crucial—is crucial I feel—for any care-person. It helped me ride those drowning waves and sustain our compassionate relationship.

Breathing mindfully in a deep way is something Robert and I practiced in earlier times when we sat down together at home to meditate. We adopted a simple teaching on mindfulness by the Vietnamese Zen Master, Thich Nhat Hanh. We silently repeated: "breathing in, I calm body and mind, breathing out, I smile. Present moment, only moment." Practicing this with Alzheimer's during tense moments with awareness present, reminded me of how precious is the moment with Robert "still here."

In spite of the trials and confusion he experienced, his tolerance and loving kindness awakened me, again and again, to a larger perspective of mind and heart, reminding me of the immediacy of each shared moment and the presence of our love. In our last years together, he became my teacher. There was no need to seek a guide elsewhere. While undergoing his own trials, he was right there with me, the most effective Zen teacher I'd ever meet.

Keeping Robert active and engaged meant driving more often in New York. We had an old Camry that wasn't too easy for him to enter and exit. The car was low and he struggled as he learned how to maneuver his long legs into the car and sit comfortably and buckle up. He enjoyed visiting the Bronxville Library located just a few minutes from his daughter's home in Westchester. We attended the regular movies and events there, but mainly Robert loved sitting on a comfortable chair in their spacious upper room reading the Times. Trusting he'd not leave the building, I'd usually take a walk or do a quick errand in the neighborhood saying, "I'll be right back."

How many times have I said that to him?

He always enjoyed coffee or tea at a cafe with a cookie. Watching others in the coffee shop, reading his paper, smiling at a toddler, enjoying the bustle of people—were treats that made his day.

We finally managed a visit to his ailing sister in New Jersey, something we hoped to do earlier, when we first arrived in New York. She lived a distance from us in the Franklin Lakes district of New Jersey, close to her son and his family. Hillary came with us on that trip to see her Aunt Betty, and volunteered to drive. This was much to my relief, as I was unfamiliar with the way.

Betty lived alone in a fine condominium, and enjoyed regular visits from her nearby son as well as her daughters, who lived in Maine, Florida, and North Carolina. When we arrived, Robert and Betty mainly reminisced about early times, his sister recounting her round-the-world trip on a Concord some years back, where "everything was taken care of"—from embarking her flight, to the hotels of her destinations, her luggage, luxurious rooms, the stupendous meals, the sightseeing and adventures she and her companions experienced, including their trip on the Orient Express. Betty's eyes sparkled as she described her journeys abroad with her children. It made Robert happy to see her thus, to see us all there together including his daughter. He didn't say much on that visit; it was enough to see his sister and daughter converse while I made tea for all of us. It was a sweet visit for him, one he dearly loved and appreciated. It was the last time he'd see Betty alive.

12

Some Political Thoughts

Sometimes less is more
but enough is always enough.
R.B.

ROBERT, 2013, NEW YORK

Politics in America is dangerously close to being taken over by corporations through their powerful lobbyists. It has been said that we are no longer the United States but Corporate States of America.

By invisible but complex control of America's wealth and resources, and by wielding the tools of merging, streamlining and down-sizing, corporations have created a materialistic aristocracy. The young become more and more aware every day of the economic and environmental lunacy they will inherit and will have to pay for.

Some corporations ignore social responsibility because they know the devious corporate secret, which is that consumerism devours the irreplaceable resources of the earth for the sake of profits. Materialism has become so mindless that it rots the humanistic fabric of everyday life.

Today, America calls for an end to political deceit and attacks between the major political parties that split the country apart. We must find common ground in order to

give America the national single-mindedness it so desper-
ately needs to resolve war, poverty, health, and education.
Only in coming together for a common good can this be
done. *Only* humanistic sensibility, not profits, will ensure
sane survival. It requires letting go of egotistical posturing
and self-centered interests and power grabs. In America,
however, knowing and accomplishing are different things.

At eighty-three I've come to see that I can seldom change
the understanding of others—only my own. A person's
understanding comes from his or her life experiences, values, and serious reflection.

We are never alone in the world. We would never survive alone. We survive only when we are aware of our inter-
connection and what can be done in this respect that will
contribute to the well-being of others.

13

"Gifts" of Alzheimer's

DIANA

I turned toward others who wrote about their own experiences with the disease to see the other side of Alzheimer's and its paradoxical gifts. Robert always pointed toward another view of things and I took him up on this. I found comfort in Joanne Koenig Coste's, *Learning to Speak Alzheimer's* and the tenets she developed while being her husband's "care partner." It helped me create a simple and easeful environment for Robert's immediate surroundings. It meant getting rid of certain furnishings and distractions that hindered his movement in the apartment.

It was always possible to communicate to Robert by paying attention to his emotions: feelings he expressed beyond words: joy, sadness, anger, contentment, a need, connection, reaching out, withdrawal. This form of communication continued to allow meaningful exchanges between us.

Feelings continue to register with people suffering from dementia even when they lose all other abilities. Sensitive response to their feelings is critical. It signals to Alzheimer's patients that they're understood and loved, that they matter, and can still communicate. Above all, it keeps them engaged daily.

Coste reminds us to encourage what a loved one with dementia can still do versus what they can no longer do.

It didn't matter that Robert could not remember the date or time or how to sign his name. He loved holding a pen or pencil and any scrap of paper he could find and would write something down even if it wasn't legible. He was still able to read a poem or an essay aloud if someone requested. We applauded him, especially when his rhythmic voice delighted us. And, when an embarrassing moment occurred through some new memory lapse, we simply ignored it and joined him in a humorous lift of the moment, appreciating his sense of humor, which, in his remaining years, became a positive aspect of his Alzheimer's journey.

Because Robert was good at camouflaging his dementia with humor especially in the mid-stages, I'd sometimes forget his situation and hold him responsible. This, however, inevitably hurt and confused him, and caused me great regret. Coste cautions never to judge, chide, or even try to reason with anyone suffering from Alzheimer's. The best possible thing was for me to join Robert, to put myself in his place, to find the joy of being with him still alive, still with me.

One can never say "I love you" often enough, especially to someone with Alzheimer's. Each moment, hearing those words, affirms their importance to us and time together. Robert said those words to me as each day passed, holding my hands. We weathered these times with words of love we both understood and I was reminded, with profound gratitude, that he was still my companion. He taught me to love what *is*.

Coste's book paved a way for me to cope with the despair and heartbreak that overwhelmed me at the most poignant of times for instance, seeing Robert struggle with buttons, his dear hands trembling. At night when he got out of bed to use the bathroom, he had a difficult time moving around the corner of his side of the bed without his glasses on. Unfortunately, I wasn't able to change this part of our furnishings. I kept a night light on but the dark of night disoriented him. I'd wake to help him as he groped his way ever so slowly around the bed. It was painful to see him struggle in what once was a natural maneuver.

There was also joy in the simple things we loved. To go for walks, meet friends in the city, exchange text and poems of our latest work, meditate. I encouraged Robert to read to me by bringing out his latest writings. When friends came, his humor naturally arose as he tried to deal with some question or statement. On the phone, when a dear friend in Portland called to say it snowed, Robert responded, "I will go to heaven, speak to God, and tell him to stop the snow for you."

In my ongoing research on Alzheimer's, I contacted ARTZ (Artists for Alzheimer's I'm Still Here Foundation) in Woburn, Massachusetts, for a copy of John Zeisel's book, *I'm Still Here*, in which he mentions the many "gifts" of Alzheimer's. Among these are new ways we establish meaningful relationships with loved ones as we learn to see the world through their eyes and appreciate the unique things that speak to them.

The gifts, as Zeisel describes, are gifts of learning to be emotionally open to others, to listen, to cherish memories;

to have a sense of humor; accept help; take care of oneself (so you may take better care of others); recognize the importance of patients' familiarity in their home, their living space, their possessions; enjoy the present; go with the flow; cope with the complicated; have a greater insight into things; learn a true sense of community, of a kinder world; to nurture, accept death, and realize the preciousness of life. These are but a few gifts in the Alzheimer's journey. The positive side of Alzheimer's is seldom mentioned. Most people think of someone with Alzheimer's as old, sick, infirmed, a person "whose mind wanders, who forgets the names of friends and family, and who is rapidly becoming a nonperson." We seldom see portrayals of someone living with the disease enjoying a concert, theater, or at a museum.

Zeisel's list of gifts experienced with Alzheimer's made me take a keener look at my own that I had divided under three "A's": Awareness, Acceptance and Appreciation—principles learned from Zen Buddhism.

Awareness encompassed everything. There was the awareness of Robert's sensitivity to voices about him. To the tones as opposed to the words used. Yet my conditioning was such that I'd often lose the clarity that comes with awareness. At times I felt like a rock needing constant running water for eons to smooth my sharp edges of delusion. The wonder of awareness showed that I was the water as well as the rock. Such times of illumination brought its many rewards, most of all, gratitude.

Acceptance was difficult. For a time, I resisted Robert's diagnosis. The struggle with denial and acceptance made me wonder about the acceptance of non-acceptance. But there was no way to avoid acceptance without imposing suffering on each other and those with whom we lived. Accepting Alzheimer's brought a realization that the only way to be effective as his care-person was to join him wholeheartedly and place myself in his skin and feel the many unpredictable trials of the disease. We learned the effective way through this path was to love *what is* in the living flow of now. To do this required placing a great faith in love, and this became the greatest teaching of all. Love that transcended all conditions or measure; love that demanded deeper, wider understanding, beyond the notion of the individual self "alone and afraid" in a world it never made.

And there was Robert's voice to appreciate. I could still coax him to read a poem or two on an afternoon when he felt particularly well, especially after dipping a cookie in a cup of English tea.

I reminded him of the time when he graduated from the Englewood School for Boys and received a hardbound copy of Whitman's *Leaves of Grass* for excellence in creative English. "You particularly liked the opening line of 'To You:'"

> Whoever you are,
> I fear you are walking the walk of dreams.

Robert looked up at me and pointed to his head, "it's all a dream," he said, "sometimes a nightmare." (He once said how he'd already learned from Edgar Alan Poe that *"all we see or seem / is but a dream within a dream."* See *Ruined Time* p. 40.) Robert was ever passionate about poetry, especially about what he knew and felt of the poetry *before* the 1950s and the poetry that came into the 1950s and produced the Beat Generation.

When I first met Robert in San Francisco, I had no clue I was meeting a Beat. I had come to him as a writer seeking help with her first novel. We were introduced by a mutual friend who worried about me spending time as a hermit on my houseboat, writing month after month on a small portable typewriter. It was 1977, before computers or Xerox machines were the norm. Robert was a literary agent who lived in an apartment on Filbert Street in the Marina district of San Francisco. I hoped he'd take me on as a client.

Living on a houseboat in Sausalito, California, I had become enamored with life floating on the water, and the natural camaraderie of neighbors who watched for the safety of my boat. I was a flight attendant at the time. My mother, who lived in Los Angeles, used to say that I was like a bird floating on the water or flying in the air and hoped I'd come down-to-earth. Somehow, writing seemed grounding.

So there I was, ringing the doorbell of a literary agent I knew very little about.

I needed help with a manuscript that had taken me over a year to write and though he did eventually help me publish a book, it wasn't the one I brought him. What I brought needed "a lot of work," Robert said kindly.

"Usually what I've found out for an aspiring writer attempting a first novel," he said, "is that it's generally a good idea to consider the first 50,000 words or so an experiment, more an exercise to maybe discard." Unfortunately, I took him literally and bravely tossed the manuscript in a trash bin by my dock when I returned home. It was the only copy I had.

Robert wore his Stetson when we went out to dine in a neighborhood restaurant on Union Street in San Francisco, sometimes forgetting he had house slippers on. Tall, handsome, with a voice made for reading prose, he would have seemed Beat to one who knew about Beats, but I knew little of the Beat Generation. My first impressions of him were of a serious writer, a lover of literature, poetry, and jazz. I remember sitting across the table at Perry's Restaurant on Union Street, talking for hours over our mutual fascination with the New Age and what it offered in higher consciousness.

Later, I was to discover the Beat element so evident and vital in him, and the humor that came naturally. With friends who knew only brand names of Beats such as Kerouac, Ginsberg or Neal Cassidy, he'd tell his own stories such as the one about Neal Cassidy who, after "mouthing off at someone, was grabbed by the shoulders of his shirt and pinned against the wall," and how Cassidy "cowered back in fear." Or, on commenting about Kerouac, "he was a very handsome guy who didn't care that he was handsome."

14

Poetry Revival in the 1950s

> ... I was drawn back into the fifties, not only
> because it was my prime time but because it had
> become an existential turning point. Never the
> product-perfect paradise some claimed, it was a
> Cold War decade of treacherous communism, of a
> horrifying hydrogen bomb, of French disasters in
> Vietnam and Algiers, and rumbles of racial rebel-
> lion throughout the South. Yet what made the fif-
> ties bearable, also made it memorable: a conscious-
> ness-changing spontaneity that came about in
> the last half of the twentieth century and sparked
> extraordinary experience. (*Ruined Time*, p. 4.)
>
> R.B.

ROBERT, 1999, OREGON,
REVISED 2012, NEW YORK

I often wonder how many people realize the incredible revival of poetry that happened in the 1950s. It was an
unusual awakening to all kinds of poets and poetry. Perhaps
the question is, Where did that revival come from and why
and how did it happen?

I believe it came about because by the end of World War
II, people were sick of lies and sick of the threats of fascism.
People were tired of propaganda and fed up with patriotic
exaggeration. In the 50s, people were hungry for honest
thought and honest speech in living language, someone saying or writing something from the heart with a true voice.

A Beat Generation emerged from a post-war interest in Yeats, Freud, Eliot, James Joyce, Picasso, Hemingway, Einstein, Gertrude Stein, Sartre, Simone de Beauvoir, and other voices from earlier times and places, voices that were rooted in Whitman, Rimbaud, and Rilke, enhanced by Dada and Surrealism, and magnified by the existentialism that ignited the consciousness of the 1950s.

15

Jazz

In the growing world of the 1940s, 1950s and 1960s, there was so much to know and always more to discover and use in order to avoid mindless living.

In 2006, my book *Ruined Time: The 1950s and the Beat*, was published. More than an autobiographical memoir, it gave a personal view of what "Beat" means and the cultural, philosophical effects of the Beat Generation in the 1950s.

To me jazz is to music what poetry is to knowing. Jazz lends an ideal combination of heart and mind as well as soul to music that in the 1950s best expressed the Beat.

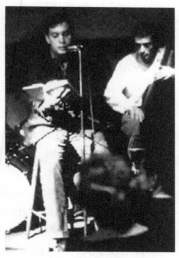

Robert reading in the Jazz Cellar, North Beach, San Francisco, CA 1959. Photograph by C. R. Snyder

Created in America, jazz was, and still is, different from other music because its sophisticated sounds impart a certain warmth and intimacy.

Jazz musicians often play the same song with variations, most of which are as thought-provoking as entertaining.

DIANA

Even as his disease progressed Robert never tired of poetry. The attempt to write a few lines of verse was ever a temptation. I remember sitting at the breakfast table, sunlight glinting on his tea cup as he held it, and asked him about poetry: could words ever express the emotions of a changing life touched by experiences with others, with nature, or the emotional relationships that affect the very depths of heart and soul? "How do we ever get a hold of a poem?"

"You can't get a poem," Robert said, "poetry has to get to you." He tried to elaborate on this thought but had difficulty recalling the right words to express his sincere feelings about writing poems.

I thought back on how he always felt a poem needed to come from the heart, from a deep passion within, a passion that continues to excite or bring joy or even suffering—to especially endure that suffering.

Then he said something about his recent attempts at poetry that touched a chord of concern and regret in him.

"I've given up on poetry," he continued. "I'm worn out now and can no longer stand or put anything on my heart. Carving is hard." But he emphasized the need for poets to "Just go—go out into the world! Write from experience!"

Robert's next reflection is drawn from that period in his past that brought such a turning point in his life.

16
The 1950s

ROBERT, 1999, OREGON,
REVISED 2012, NEW YORK

The 1950s were a fountainhead of prosperity and promise. Looking back, however, it was also a period in which modern times were betrayed by an undertow of cultural and political duplicity. It was an era of seductive consumption but demanding conformity. A trying period in which limits of human potential were being ruthlessly revised by artists, writers, poets, and humanists of every stripe.

What the Beat did was to magnify and intensify the American experience—to revise forms and values and rack them with a kind of sweet but crazed seriousness that often swept poetry out of universities and into the streets.

Even today, modern poetry deals with answers to questions that have not been asked—with feelings that have not been experienced—which is why poetry disturbs us so. In being disturbed, we are often inspired, and by being inspired, something new, something unimaginable invades our minds.

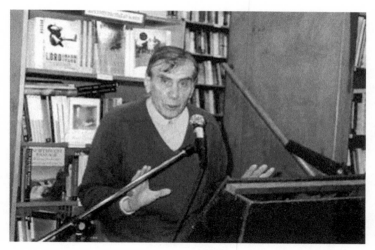

Robert at Borders Bookstore, Portland, OR, 2003. Photo by Diana Saltoon

William Carlos Williams said, "It is difficult to get the news from poems, yet people die miserable deaths every day for lack of what is found there."

Beat writers, all of whom developed a certain seeing, helped me see that for all of the technological wonder upon which I had become so dependent something was and is still not right in America. Why is it that even today—in an age of spectacular information—we still buy into the same old myth that science can solve everything. Isn't it pathetic that we still ignore what the anthropologist Loren Eiseley wrote in 1961—that science was "as capable of decay as any human activity such as religion or any system of government."

The best Beat poetry, like the best Beat art, opened insight into everything.

17

The Beat Phenomenon

ROBERT, 2011, NEW YORK

In the larger scheme of things, life turns toward terrains of kinder concern and giving. Perhaps returning to what began in my time—the late 1940s and 1950s—the Beat phenomenon, with its welcome shadows hardly seen but felt then, can bring calm to receptive hearts.

The Beat phenomenon was a creative change expressed in lifestyles, music and literature that was and is anti-establishment and always relaxed. That the Beat phenomenon has been kept alive is shown by the fact that Jack Kerouac's book *On the Road* has not been out of print since 1957. Among other things, the book represents the individual freedom of going anywhere—at any time.

The only time I ever saw and spoke with Jack Kerouac was in San Francisco in 1959. He was with Lew Welch and Albert Saijo outside of the Jazz Workshop, where they were getting ready to drive to New York. My conversation with Kerouac was brief, but despite the amount of alcohol in him, I was more than impressed with his style of telling me how and why they were going to New York. As Kerouac talked to me, I listened to a man I would never forget. That Beat man opened my mind to a wider vision in which harmony existed side by side with adversity. Yet, as any Beat would say, "It's possible. Anything's possible! Why not?"

Larger visions bring us to a level of understanding of how deep our interdependence on one another is. It's then that it is possible to see more than is seen—even become more than we are, which leads to a greater consciousness. There is more to the lives we are living, such as being freed from a mindless existence that concentrates only on basic survival and a worship of materialism.

DIANA

Although Robert only took a "toke" now and then in San Francisco, as it was sparingly available then, we had one experience together with Psilocybin, something a friend gave when Robert and I first met and spent time together on my houseboat.

The day we shared the Psilocybin on my houseboat, Robert guided me throughout the experience taking care of my journey with the drug. With him, I felt safe, cherished and nurtured. It wasn't an earthshaking experience, except seeing Robert in his blue sweater as a spiral of brilliant energy swirls and his eyes as two luminous pools of turquoise. All my senses however, were keenly attuned—to the call of a gull, the scent of the salty air, the tactile feel of the shawl Robert had placed on my shoulders or the lunch we had later in a restaurant in Tiburon where they served giant shrimps with delectable sauce. Each sensation was magnified with feelings of expansion, benevolence, and charm. Even the flotsam off the dock of the restaurant seemed a thing of beauty and delight. The sound of laughter from a nearby group of rowdy kids off their parents' boat brought laughter to my own heart and giggles when Robert shoved a shrimp into my mouth.

At eighty-three years, the only drugs he now takes are small doses of Galantamine and Memantine to help slow the progress of his disease, but they seem more of a placebo.

18

A Psychedelic Experience

> The 1950s opened another door that revealed that
> only a real use of drugs leads away from drugs.
>
> R.B.

ROBERT, 1983, CALIFORNIA,

REVISED 2014, OREGON

One of my most memorable experiences during the 1950s was driving down the Pacific Coast and taking a trip up into the wondrous wilds of Big Sur, California, where I camped with four other Korean War veterans and discovered mescaline, which opened up levels of seeing.

We were a small band of young and older men who met at Big Sur and hopped in a Mercury station wagon together to take a trip to the Garapata Creek. But we found ourselves south of that and already south of the Sierra Creek as well. So we filled five canteens from a hose behind a restaurant, piled into the car, and drove back a few miles before peeling off onto a higher Coast Road then on a single dirt lane where we found a place to park.

There the hood was lifted on the wagon and a couple of ignition wires toyed with after the back end was opened. We took turns pocketing matches and shaking out big, scruffy pieces of khaki oilcloth to sleep on. In that shuffle I noticed that one dude had a Colt .45 tucked in a well-oiled holster, but I didn't say anything. By then it seemed that what would happen already had. Circles of thick and thin trees ushered us along a winding, uphill hike. Criss-crossing a couple of grades, we high-stepped over the bubbling of a couple of small streams.

An hour later, after nodding over a sheltered meadow, we settled down to eat and pass joints while waiting out the night.

For hours I laid and watched the stars decorate patches of sky until, beginning to doze, I suddenly worried about where I'd hidden the key after I locked my door on Telegraph Hill in San Francisco. For fear of losing it, I hadn't brought it along. But, before I could panic, the moving black and green hues of the chilly woods flushed such silence through the brush that there was no longer any key, or door.

We woke up to trickling water and songs of Steller jays, red-tailed hawks, and maybe even the spiraling spirit of an invisible condor. When it was light enough, pieces of cheese and pizza bread were passed around, then a couple of canteens while the taller dude smoothed a corner of his oilcloth and emptied out a rumpled sack of half-dried brown-crinkled mushrooms that looked like warped Civil War buttons. As if with foxhole efficiency, he scraped off inner circles of tiny but prickly barbs. The longer he slit and rearranged the pile, the more he whetted the anticipation of something ancient, of vile swallows that fouled the mouth with bitter but desirable bile. However, after all of this was passed, my brain and mind began to spill out of my head and recreate a gigantic lost heart-magic that seemed to undo old worlds and prolong a roll of beautifully colored wonder in which trees hanged greens and shapes while some mothering heaven softly rippled endless patterns of feeling over the earth. The beauty of sensation was beyond splendor, and being so subjective, so solitary, it defied description or measure. For what seemed like endlessly melted minutes but were actually ten or fifteen hours, I struggled to use and not be used by the narcotic's change of the visually bloated but beautiful nature around me; the uncertainty of mysteriously different nomenclature that was revealed in the higher wings of trees, the elbows of clouds and elegant waves of grass. Undulating grass that bordered an unending spread of moss and sunlight and darkness in which the music of the wind and flows of elusive water were captured around and then down in front of a countless mix of phantom memories. Memories that glowed like the microscopic head pools that filled so many of my hands while soaking my changing faces with an unimaginable glint of that first awesome light of Christ. A light that flooded my soul before I could tell myself that I'd never be the same, ever, because I'd glimpsed the meaning of stars.

Ambling down Big Sur was a baffling descent that led us back to the old Coast Road where the muddy hood of the station wagon creaked when it was lifted. Once the ignition was reconnected and the car backed around toward Nepenthe Restaurant no one said a word. The parking lot seemed alien, weird to us. We quickly de-grouped and paused with our backs to the ocean in order to flash knowing nods to one another before driving away.

19

Anniversary

DIANA

ANNIVERSARY

Where to begin?
Each day I awake
to find you near,
loving, kind,
forgiving, giving
My day begins
nourished
like this: your forgiveness
untarnished, pure.
Not thinking
how it will be
when you're no longer here,
when the well of love
I drink from is gone.

D.S.

When I met Robert at his apartment in San Francisco armed with my ill-fated novel, the moment I stepped into his living room, I fell in love with it. At the time, I had a propensity for falling in love with men where they lived, as when my first husband invited me to his home at Incline Village, to what he called his "cabin" overlooking a ski slope. Later, after our divorce, I met a photographer and film-maker who lived in a tented camp on the

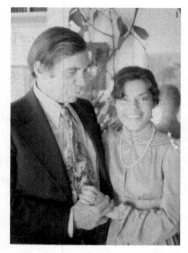

Robert and Diana, December, 1979, in their apartment on Filbert Street, San Francisco, CA. Photo by Jean Woods

Serengeti Plains of East Africa where I dearly wanted to live. I was also interested in photography and was intrigued by the idea of studying and photographing animals in the wild. So, for six months, I ended up living in that tented camp on the Serengeti Plains.

Living in the African wilds turned out to be a phenomenal turning point in my life; after that I was never quite the same again. The natural lifestyle we led on the Serengeti seemed the most human way to live. It brought a compassionate understanding of impermanence and the intrinsic connection I shared with all of life and nature. The cycle of life and death was vividly evident in the continuous activity of creation and destruction around us and in the natural activity of the predators and the hunted. However, the surroundings in the wild—the unending sky, the wide and beautiful vistas—didn't guarantee a husband and lasting relationship, so I eventually returned home to San Francisco, single, but with a new interest—exploring words this time. Fortunately, my interest in words and writing led to Robert and what became an enduring relationship of love and friendship.

Robert's two-bedroom apartment in the Marina district of San Francisco was far from luxurious, adventurous, or large, but well appointed. The living room had a warm, welcome feel that encircled you with its friendly presence. There was a marble mantelpiece above a working fireplace, long bookshelves filled with books by interesting authors I wanted to meet, a tall lamp with soft light by a black leather couch, a writing desk to the side of the room, and, against a wall, a high, long, useful desk which was obviously used for book projects. Moving towards the bookshelves, I recognized names of authors such as Doug Boyd, who wrote about the American Indian medicine man Rolling Thunder, and Jack Schwartz, the famous Dutch psychic who had confounded Elmer and Alyce Green at the Menninger Foundation in Topeka, Kansas when they hooked him up to biofeedback. There was Kenneth Pelletier, PhD, author of *Mind as Healer, Mind as Slayer,* who had been featured in a workshop I had just attended called "The Mind Can Do Anything," and Arthur Middleton Young, the inventor of the Bell Helicopter who had written *The Reflexive Universe* and founded the Institute for the Study of Consciousness in Berkeley, California. Robert had helped each of them with their manuscripts and successfully had them published.

I instinctively thought, "Here's a man who's a conduit to knowledge."

Seated in his living room on the comfortable couch as Robert offered me a glass of wine and took my manuscript box, I felt I never wanted to leave the place. But I was there on business—or so I thought.

The truth was I fell in love with the way Robert had made San Francisco his home. The way he loved the city and all it stood for at the time—a place where art and free expression were as much a part of the city as its hills, sunshine, rain and fog, ocean and bridges. A place that inspired his poem: *Time and San Francisco.*

20

Time and San Francisco

ROBERT, 2012, NEW YORK

TIME AND SAN FRANCISCO

Time is immaterial in San Francisco.
It's an ageless city from the sky,
but once you've matched the moan of a fog-horn
with more than one unexpected streetlight
you know you'll never be quite the same
unless you stay or
every year or so
admit you have to return.

Some believe veiled sweeps of spirits
flow east from the ocean.
These begin in the north
below Mendocino and
down south just above Big Sur
before haunting skyscrapers
and vanishing in the towering sequoias
high in the Sierra Nevada mountains.

Such fables beguile you for a while.
But they're bound to bewitch and
weeks or years later,
generate a smoldering loneliness
that numbs the imagination and
exposes your soul to
what you were in
San Francisco.

R.B.

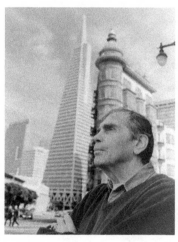

Robert, North Beach, San Francisco,
CA, 1999. Photo by Mark Eifert

21

A Dewdrop World

DIANA

A DEWDROP WORLD

Dewdrops appear perfectly
reflecting the whole world
then disappear as moments do
containing everything
lived or not lived.

D.S.

Turning beyond eighty-three found Robert at another
stage in Alzheimer's where, even as he steadily lost the ability to converse, he still reflected and celebrated aging.

In New York in 2013, writing had become increas-
ingly difficult and so Robert turned to his care-person for
help. Rosemary, who arrived and allowed me to do errands
or keep an appointment, dutifully typed words on a computer for Robert as he struggled to remember, helping him

along the way. But it frustrated him when she tried to edit mid-way, before his sentences were done. Both carried on, as best as they could and waited for me to return and soothe what misunderstandings occurred.

22

Thoughts on Aging

ROBERT, 2013, NEW YORK

Often some people are aging and do not know it—for various reasons. They're aging but they are holding on to youth without being aware of it. This is unfortunate because everyone needs to be aware of aging and its changes. We need to realize such effects and need to be aware that different people live different lives.

Elders are coming to the end of life, an end of living. It's painful to face decline and loss. Exercise *does* help. However, the older people grow, the more difficulties they encounter and have to come to terms with.

Even so-called "uniform" aging differs in men and women or even people of the same gender. People's individual responses to their aging differ as well. Those who ignore obvious signs of aging, which others would *not* ignore, are in danger of things becoming significantly worse for them. In other words, we have to *pay attention* to our own self and what it's telling us. Never think that taking care of the self, "taking it easy," is wrong or self-indulgent. Even taking care of the "self" varies in aged people.

We have to be wise about what we can and cannot do—and should or should not do. Just because others do outstanding things does not mean that we should do them. Once again, we have to listen to the inner self.

23

Positive Aspects of Aging

ROBERT, 2013, NEW YORK

There are some *wonderful* aspects to aging—feelings of accomplishment and fulfillment, maturity and wisdom, and perspective on one's life—as well as other people's too, and, if one is very blessed, having achieved the "true love" that was once hoped for in youth.

I never believed I would pass eighty years, let alone eighty-three. Now, all these days leave me with a deep love and thanks to my family, my daughter, my wife, and to years of wonderful friends—each of whom were with me, and occasionally saved me from some mindless consideration of what I was trying to do.

For me what has become important is to notice the precious moments given in life, in that blue sky that seems bluer wherever I am.

24

Winter Memories

ROBERT, 2013, NEW YORK

As I gaze out the window on a lovely winter day, with grounds white from a recent beautiful snow, I am reminded of unforgettable memories of past winters with family and friends.

When I was a boy during the Depression, I remember being pulled on sleighs, which were thrilling to slide off of, and running to look through shiny red, green, and gold frosted windows, which seemed to radiate brighter and brighter, especially in the years of the Depression.

During those years, my father was fortunate in that he had steady employment with the Omaha Power and Light Company. And so, our family at least, had shelter and was never hungry.

DIANA

Sometimes the circumstances of early life so carve into our being that they almost become DNA within our cells and atoms, as when, for example, I was born in Singapore during World War II and loud bombs hit the island, demolishing life and buildings. So much so that, throughout my life, there remained the residue of fear in the presence of armed militia. Robert's early life was greatly influenced by the Great Depression that began in 1929, the year he was born. The atmosphere he experienced of great need and suffering deeply imprinted his consciousness.

25
Together

DIANA

TOGETHER

How many days and months?
Silly to count time like this when
each moment is just right
as it comes and goes
in your encircling warmth
that's always present
even in times of stress.

No words.
This deep gratitude,
blessed with your love
unconditional as it is.
only this:
to hold you
knowing life's fragility.

D.S.

Our life in San Francisco took many turns. We moved out of the apartment in the Marina District when Robert lost his lease and needed another place. For a time, there was a studio space on the upper floor of Arthur Young's Institute for the Study of Consciousness in Berkeley, where we stored books and conducted business while commuting from my houseboat.

It was also a time when Robert produced a series of Broadside Editions based on Young's earlier works, *The Reflexive Universe* and *The Geometry of Meaning*. A series of moves led us to Lucas Valley and then Corte Madera in Marin County, where we found rentals that were reasonable and areas that encouraged walking. Robert had a core of male friends—he called his "Praetorian Guards"—close companions who loved hiking in the Marin hills and out by Point Reyes, the highlight of their walk being a lunch or dinner later at a gourmet restaurant in Marin County or San Francisco, where they felt justified in eating well and having fine wine or beer. When one of the "guards" passed away unexpectedly, they continued to toast his memory at their gourmet ventures and kept their friendship alive long after the rigorous hikes were over and Robert and I moved away.

We relocated to Portland, Oregon in the spring of 1990. Our initial impression of Portland was that of a friendly town, a kindly town, rather forgiving in many ways, as Robert said.

We bought a house in Portland, something we couldn't afford to do in San Francisco; a home with enough rooms for our small business. We helped authors ready their books for publishing with the help of our associates, a loose-knit group of writers, editors and book designers. Our family room had glass doors that opened to a deck with a lovely garden that invited tranquility.

In Portland we joined Zen meditation groups and I continued my practice in the Japanese Way of Tea. Robert connected with new writers, publishers, editors, photographers and musicians. Our circle of friendship in Oregon steadily expanded. Robert had a close friend who had moved from San Francisco to the Oregon coast and owned a bookstore. In 1990 Robert dedicated a poem to his friend.

26

On The Beach at Cannon Beach

ROBERT, 1990, OREGON

(for John)

ON THE BEACH AT CANNON BEACH

Before the big bald rock
Big Sur is still south of San Francisco
and New York's east of Mount Hood.

Up here, I wonder if in some forgotten room
you're not waiting to explain why
scenes always ended once we discovered
that in the poetry of lush love
whatever was found was lost.

And I wonder if different jazz
still inspires that last lonely woman
to turn as if
her shadow perfumes the wall
and disturbs the lean listener
who fingers
a disconnected telephone.

                                    R.B.

27

The Way Within

DIANA

THE WAY WITHIN

The way within
goes through the body
blood, veins, muscles,
bones, organs,
to relax deeper
through partially opened eyes
to sink into cells and atoms
and let go
until just breath
guiding breath
then almost no
breath.

Stillness and space open
when the mind of no mind
becomes a hushed awareness
in empty space
no body seen

just the slightest
breeze of breath
in vast silence
with subtle sounds arising
disappearing, arising again
in the universe of awareness.

D.S.

In our Oregon home in the early 1990s, we continued with Robert's publishing business, hoping to establish our Broadside Editions and other books. Before Arthur Young's death in 1995, Robert went back and forth to Berkeley working with Arthur on new publications. Robert had a great love and admiration for him. Arthur was a kind of mentor, a man of brilliant intellect and

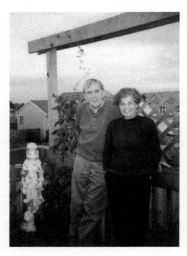

Robert and Diana in Oregon, 2004.
Photo by Ted Bagley

genius. An American inventor who created the stabilizer bar for helicopters and designed the Bell Helicopter, Young was also a cosmologist, philosopher, and keen astrologer. He believed in the Theory of Process, an integral theory of human thought and experience. He incorporated science and physics into his theory but went beyond science. To him the universe couldn't be limited to physical measurement. Young embraced the concept of "a great chain of being" and influenced many thinkers of the time, such as Fritjof Capra and Stanislav Grof, to name a few.

As members of the Zen Center of Oregon, I eventually took the Buddhist precepts and became lay-ordained, but Robert stayed just outside the circle, observing and absorbing, in an existential way, his own understanding of Zen. He'd say to me, whenever I urged him to join me on a weekday meditation with the Zen group in the city, "you go ahead and sit with them today, I'll sit here at home instead." His "sitting" was a prone position on the floor, what he called meditation in the yogic pose of "the dead man asana." However, he did occasionally sit with the group, enjoying the camaraderie of friends and caring people.

28

Zen

ROBERT, 2011, OREGON

I've found Zen meditation extraordinarily helpful. On different levels it offers a spiritual and psycho-physiological way to wellness. Zen profoundly points to that intrinsic connection we have with all beings and nature. The realization of being interdependent brings a clear need for integration—not separation. This is more than ever necessary as we move forward in a new millennium.

In the growing freedom of creativity, the healing space of silence, we discover who and what we are, why we need to act in awareness—an awareness in which we free ourselves to heed spiritual and ecological demands. This is the heart of understanding in which we experience the truth that, in today's world, we are never alone.

Meditation opened my eyes to that larger view of reality that ultimately expresses a natural compassion for each other and all living beings.

As I become more familiar with the benefits and tranquility of Zen, I am better able to remember where I have

come from and what I have done and how I might continue
a richer life.

It has inspired me to write this poem:

THE ZEN OF SEEING

High in the mind's sky
rolling mandala clouds rise
out of the darkness of mystery and
from those shadows comes light and
out of light comes life.
Even modern science agrees with that.
And out of life comes love,
and out of love comes understanding,
and from understanding comes equanimity.
Science doesn't notice that.
Equanimity is the level on which
we see why
the opposite of understanding is chaos—
why the opposite of love is hate.
why the opposite of life is death and
why the opposite of light is mystery
and darkness again—until
out of the level of equanimity comes
compassion—and from compassion comes
the freedom of forgiveness.
Forgiveness is the level of great
expectations—it is that level of
independence in which we begin to
see more than is seen
know more than is learned and
become more than we are.

We see how awareness leads to greater
consciousness and that larger
life in which we profit from
purpose and the benefit of acceptance.
And realize that the lives we lead
we have led before—and will lead again
as women—as men—wise or foolish—
cruel or kind—rich or poor—powerful or weak—
black—red—brown—white—or yellow—
life after life—we
revolve in and out of the
endless mystery and dark.
And as wise Zen Master Dogen says
"being enlightened does not divide—
Just as the moon does not break the water."
This Zen of seeing cannot be hindered.
Just as a drop of water
reflecting the moon
does not hinder the moon in the sky
the Zen of seeing leads to that
kinder terrain of caring in a deep way
where the cycle of giving and receiving
is ever wide and continuous.

R.B.

29

Another Birthday

DIANA

Another birthday
another celebration of life.
Seeing your dear face, your smile
as you raise your morning tea
still steaming while—
you take stock of the day
I want to say many things—
express my happiness for you and—
how to—how to—express
the inexpressible gratitude
that rises with this simple
thank you!

D.S.

The year was 2001, a full decade before Alzheimer's entered our minds. I had given this poem to Robert on his birthday in June, three months before the 9/11 terrorist attacks. We had moved from our Oregon City home outside

Portland into a new house we purchased in Scappoose, Oregon, about thirty minutes from NW Portland.

September 11, 2001 changed all our lives.

To heal the shattered confidence of a "safe" America, some of us thought of ways to meet and create a meaningful communion a month after the attack. Our dear friends invited us along with others to a potluck gathering at their home that we might share our thoughts and feelings about the disaster.

For me, the experience of *Chanoyu*, as in the Way of Tea, never failed to bring harmony and peace into the hearts of participants. So, we proposed a moon-viewing tea for the event. Our friends lived close to the Willamette River and had an exquisite garden and deck that made a perfect spot for an outdoor tea gathering.

That night, guests were each served sweets and a bowl of whisked green tea beneath a full moon lighting the garden. The temperature was mild for a late October evening, a slight breeze stirring the cherry tree, beneath which we placed a tatami mat and our utensils for making tea. A candle lit the iron kettle and the maroon lacquered tea box. The moon glowed on our friends' faces, reflecting calm and beauty of the night garden and our simple ceremony.

Afterwards, we adjourned indoors and shared poems and stories that helped bring trust, caring, and connection back to our hearts that had been lost in a country changed by sudden, cruel circumstances.

Robert wrote a short piece for the event.

30

On the Tragedy of September 11, 2001

ROBERT, 2001, OREGON

In times like these—when death and fear and trouble seem to overwhelm us—it's wise that we come together to recover roots of friendship and renewal, wise that we touch and look to one another for the support and understanding we all need. In times like these, I look back—back into poetry, because good poetry offers rare relief that is hard to find.

So, in times like these, we should look for that which helps us see and believe, that no matter what the crisis, there's always a way to restore that vital air of introspection that cleanses the mind. Always a way to create some sanctuary of removal and understanding in which it is possible to recover the spirit of being and that root-heart of America.

Looking back, I found insights that sobered my perspective and found a poem by Carl Sandburg that more than comforted me.

In 1945 Henry Miller wrote *The Air-Conditioned Night-mare*, and in it he said:

> It isn't the oceans that cut us
> off from the rest of the world
> —it's the American way
> of looking at things.

In 1920 Carl Sandburg wrote a magnificent poem called *Haze*:

> Keep a red heart of memories
> under the great grey rain sheds of sky,
> under the open sun
> and the yellow gloaming embers.
> Remember all paydays of lilacs and songbirds;
> all starlights of cool memories on storm paths . . .
> (FROM THE COLLECTION
> *Smoke and Steel*, 1920)

DIANA

Post 9/11, Robert continued to look to poetry, the Beat, and jazz to inspire him in an America so changed and still changing—but not, he felt, for the better.

In 2006, Robert's book, *Ruined Time: The 1950s and the Beat*, was published. Previous to that, Robert did a CD— *Poetry and the 1950s: Homage to the Beat Generation*, inspired by the book. Both were works based on his love of poetry and the jazz that came with and off of it.

According to a review from poet and Beat, David Melt-zer, "*Ruined Time*, is a book within the book, the history within the mystery, the mythology of the '50s, the so-called Beat Generation. Briggs reveals the real deal as a participant in that confounding history. His work is a remarkable embodiment of the personal as the political; a brave demonstration of tough insight, survival, and triumph. Briggs brings it all into play—not as a fantasy or mythoblathering hype, but as the ongoing and complex struggle all dissident spirits had to (and have to) contend with in dark yet illuminated days."

In the early stages of Alzheimer's, prior to the diagnosis, Robert began a series of reads on Jazz and Poetry & Other Reasons.

31

Jazz and Poetry & Other Reasons

ROBERT, 2013, NEW YORK

My interest in jazz and poetry grew in 2008 when, with the help of my wife, I began a successful series of "reads" we titled *Jazz and Poetry & Other Reasons*. Most of these reads were accompanied by a jazz trio composed of friends I'd known a long while.

For several years I performed reads accompanied with the trio in various venues in Portland. The reads were based on *Ruined Time: The 1950s and the Beat.*

These combinations of poetry with jazz were so successful that I continued to write and perform them with the musicians until the fall of 2011 when my wife and I moved to New York. In New York, I hoped to continue performing reads to jazz.

We called the reads "Opuses." The first in the series is *Opus One: The Beat Goes On*, a blend of poetry and music that deals with the Beat belief that there is "more to life than living." There is "seeing more than is seen, knowing more than is learned, and becoming more than you are."

The next in the series, *Opus Two: Love in America: from Romanticism to Globalism*, describes four very different American poets, Edgar Allan Poe, Carl Sandburg, Kenneth Patchen, and Sharon Olds. Edgar Allan Poe's tragic luck; Carl Sandburg's belief that modern history was just a "bucket of ashes;" Kenneth Patchen's dark poetry, that of a social protest poet, an accomplished artist, as well as a highly original poet.

Sharon Olds, a politically liberal poet, has an unusual feminine touch to her poetry and she adds a taste of modern jazz to her work. Olds' work deals with individual, political, and literary reaction to the huge events of the day.

> . . . many women of the world
> who took options out on Sharon Olds'
> *Sex Without Love* were either pioneers
> or compulsive erotics
> or part of a growing number of guiltless romantics
> who floated the same ways and means
> of free freedom that the Beat Generation
> came to believe in . . .
>
> R.B.

In today's America, romanticism hardly has a history and globalism seems to have—at best—an uncertain future in which only the lonely survive.

Sharon Olds carries her readers beyond the status quo of almost everything.

Opus Three: Homage to the Beat Generation traces the roots of the Beat movement following its rise in Greenwich Village, New York, through to North Beach, San Francisco, to Paris, France, and many points in-between, creating an atmosphere in which we can feel the breath of change and hear the echo of footsteps heading towards the door.

Opus Four, Zen and the Kerouac Curse takes a keen look at Jack Kerouac, his work, his fascination with Zen Buddhism, the continuous effect of American Zen on the Beat persuasion, and his demise due to alcoholism.

> ... *On the Road* is a book once read
> reminds the serious reader that
> America is continually cursed
> by the inflated demands of materialism
> that haunts—not only the existentialist
> but the spirit of the Beat and the Outsider
> who were and are still willing and able
> to do whatever is necessary
> to create new ways to greater freedom
> and that sane integration that reveals
> the keys to those rights and wrongs
> that offer new and better ways
> to discover many long and short roads
> to individual freedom ...
>
> R.B.

The next, *Opus Five, The Best Minds*, deals with "the best minds of our generation" who not only struggle with worldwide depressions but also with the changes coming in and out of the Obama presidency which seem to raise some endless glow of hope over what has and is still being harried by political deceit. In Ginsberg's *Howl*, we see that

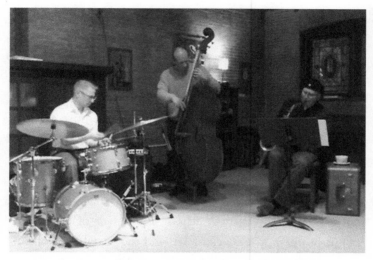

Jazz trio accompanying Robert, TaborSpace, Portland, OR, 2010. Stuart
Fessant on Sax, Dan Davis on bass, and Tim DuRoche on drums.
Photo by Chel White

the "best minds" of those
who were saying "no" to
the sad and mad material-
ism of the 1950s—and then
too often saying "yes" to
that birth-controlled magic
of the 1960s. We can only
hope that these same minds
would emerge over the next
half a century to say "NO"
to the present, insidious
growing class of an American materialistic aristocracy
choking the middle class to
death.

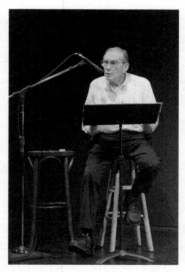

Robert reading with his jazz trio at
TaborSpace, Portland, OR, 2010.
Photo by Mark Eifert

Other reads from Jazz and Poetry & Other Reasons include *Opus Six: Why the Beat Haunts the American Mind*, a discussion about the continuing attraction of the Beat to the American public, long after the 1950s. Of course, the big names in the Beat movement were Kerouac, Ginsberg, Burroughs, and Corso. There is always far more to know about the Beat effect of those lost idealists, those haunted and haunting souls who are usually remembered by people.

Without deepening awareness of consciousness, we do not live, we only exist. Without the power of poetry, the magic of music, the shock of art, and the visual logic of film, we never cross frontiers of understanding—or reach summits of equanimity and compassion, we do not inquire, we do not grow, and we end up stagnated.

Arthur Young once said that consciousness is "what you need when things don't work!"

Why does the Beat haunt the American mind? Of course, the Beat myth is an historical link with the 1950s—not only because of the Beat effect on American consciousness but because what the Beats feared back then is what the young now dread. That is the problem of materialism, often at the expense of humanity, which can become a drag on true democracy.

Why does the Beat still haunt the American mind—when those 1950s were hardly idyllic?

The nostalgia for the Beat Generation reveals the need to get back into saner climates and recognitions that remind us that the lives we lead need far more than power or wealth. They need to be recognized and shadowed by kind words and music and by the poetry of jazz and the jazz of poetry.

The Beat accentuated an enormous interest in existentialism: "Man is nothing else but what he makes of himself."

With mindful action, we create a more meaningful reality in which we establish purpose in our lives. Purpose is the key with which we free ourselves and heed spiritual and ecological imperatives which are the heart of the Beat inheritance.

Opus Seven: The Beat Returns is a mix of facts and memories that take us back to the 1950s and the Beat, to poetry that crosses time and politics and various ways of the heart. Ways that lead to trust and a kinder terrain where those who trailed other loners out of doors or down streets did so in order to see and be more and come to keener understanding. To see that jazz was indeed to music what poetry was to knowing. Knowing that came from a love of poetry that addressed not only growing environmental concerns but the politics of the times, the shared love of nature and human possibilities. All of which is connected with a freedom that goes beyond and above fear or aggression and deception. Above all, beyond the propaganda of negative voices that poisons the American mind.

The last of the *Jazz and Poetry & Other Reasons* series, *Opus Eight: The Beat Revealed,* written in June of 2011, attempts to answer the question of why, after so many decades, the Beat continues to haunt the American mind by shedding a critical light on present-day America, a nation that in the turn of the 21st Century, seems to flounder at its very foundation—democracy and the pursuit of happiness for all.

> . . . what I have learned in the way
> of life is that there is always a way
> always a way out of trouble or anxiety
> so long as there is faith in life and
> trust in the larger flow of life held
> by a mind wider than the sky
> clear and unhindered . . .
> There is a heartbeat I can steady
> when I open to acceptance and trust
> a beat with a rhythm of its own and
> I can appreciate that rhythm for
> it brings another moment to breathe
> to live, to love and, above all to be loved.
>
> R.B.

32

Change

DIANA

CHANGE

The certainty in
uncertainty
the permanence
of impermanence
inseparable with change
as in a shadow—
my shadow—
yours
shifting
in moving light
change
moment by moment now.

D.S.

Robert came home a little late one day, carrying a bag of groceries he'd bought in town after an afternoon appointment with a literary friend.

I remember he was backlit by the afternoon sun as I came down the stairs. He greeted me and held me longer than usual, before he sat me on the couch.

"Something wrong?" I asked.

He shook his head.

But he took my hand and turned to face me. "I need to tell you something."

"Yes?" Something in his voice made me apprehensive.

"On my way home I pulled over and turned the engine off and sat in the car because I couldn't go on. To tell the truth, I was lost."

"What happened?"

"I couldn't remember where I was or where I was going."

Alarmed, I took his hand. "Why didn't you call?"

"I don't remember. I must have forgotten to take the phone. Took some time before I realized I was driving home."

I held him close. "You're here, thank goodness." For a long time I worried about the incident. I hoped it was a passing one, just a minor memory lapse.

It was summer, 2009. Within the past year he'd had two operations, one of them serious.

After his car incident, I paid keener attention and noticed other signs that concerned me. His struggle to speak spontaneously in interviews, or answer questions after giving a talk unless he read off written answers to specific questions—something he'd never done earlier. More and more, he left our publishing business and finances for me to handle (something questionable at best), although I didn't mind taking care of our bills, checks, and correspondence. A close friend noticed that Robert was not as lively engaged as he normally was when we got together at her home and wondered if there was something wrong. When I mentioned his memory lapse, she recommended Aricept, a drug her father took that helped with his memory.

I made an appointment for a consultation with Robert's primary care doctor. After a brief neurological test, she mentioned "signs of slight dementia" and prescribed a light dose of Galantamine Hydrobromide, similar to Aricept. I did not know it was also used for Alzheimer's Disease. "Having Alzheimer's"—never entered our minds.

The financial strain we were experiencing at the time must have certainly added to Robert's condition, especially after we lost the equity in our home. However, he was still able to drive and continued to write and perform his jazz and poetry readings—which kept him alert and very engaged. I especially encouraged his performances to keep his memory alive. The 1950s were a formulating time, a period in his life when literature took such a keen hold of him and guided his life.

We finally sold our home. It was 2011 and we were moving to New York that fall. The thought of seeing his daughter again enlivened Robert and the activities of our move inspired him with plans to introduce his reads to New York college campuses.

In New York, however, we could no longer ignore Robert's growing memory lapses nor his doctor's diagnosis of Alzheimer's. Yet, New York opened other avenues for us. In spite of his Alzheimer's diagnosis, Robert loved New York, where he hoped to continue reading and writing. We met a young woman whose father had recently passed away from Alzheimer's and she understood Robert's condition with empathy and love. Besides, she was a lover of poetry and music and wherever and whenever she could, supported her many friends in the performing arts. We became close friends. She introduced us to a club in Manhattan, where she encouraged Robert to participate in literary Open Mic events held once a month at the club's library. We met other performing artists, comedians, musicians, actors, directors, and writers. It was a stimulating time and kept Robert and me from the depression and anxiety of his progressing memory loss.

* * *

2013. Robert's participation in a clinical trial had ended and there wasn't another for him. In a short time, his situation worsened. Sometimes he'd point his hand to his head and say "What's happening? What's this?" He rarely showed frustration, but when he did, my heart broke from not being able to halt the disease. He could still read somewhat, but writing and conversing became difficult. To counteract his inability to answer direct questions, he'd come back with amusing remarks such as, "I gave up on remembering."

Or, when talking about microphones, "had one so strong a line of ants across a table sounded like horses." Or on Bill O'Reilly, "he gives bullshit a whole new odor."

Or, when I asked, "Briggs what are you truly feeling?"

"Life," he answered.

Sometimes I called Robert—"Briggs." I don't know why except through the years of knowing him, the name "Briggs," seemed to lend itself naturally when addressing

him much as "Bob" did, although if you asked what he pre-
ferred to be called, he'd say "Robert." But he never minded
whether you called him Robert, Briggs, or Bob, as he'd
answer gladly to all three.

His wit never deserted him. It endured even as his memory kept fading. One night, while we drove with a friend
through Manhattan, we were overcome by the view of the
city. Our friend and I enthusiastically commented on how
magical it looked—the skyscrapers, the sidewalks, the sights
and lights of the city beneath a full moon on "such a clear
night!"

Robert just said, "It's New York."

As much as Briggs hoped to give reads on campuses, we
knew that wasn't an option anymore. Even though he still
had a captivating voice, it was difficult to answer questions
from an audience.

At the club in Manhat-
tan, however, Robert found
an opportunity to read what
he so passionately loved—
sharing his thoughts about
the Beat era. He was introduced as a "Beat poet,"
even though he never con-
sidered himself "Beat," or
a poet. However, he made
his way to the microphone
and shared the recent prose
he wrote in 2013, two years
after his diagnosis.

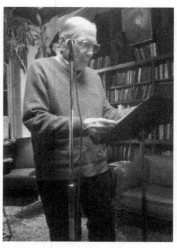

Robert reading at The Players in
Manhattan, NY, 2012. Photo by
Craig Pravda

33

A Return to Greenwich Village

ROBERT, 2013, NEW YORK

A RETURN TO GREENWICH VILLAGE

In 2013, mine is a glazed return
to Greenwich Village where back
in 1950 I first sold books
at the Eighth Street and Marlboro Bookstores
and listened to jazz in the Five Spot and
sat in the White Horse Tavern on Hudson Street
watching Dylan Thomas drink himself to death
before I took another subway back
up to the West End Bar and Grill where
I knew funky rooms were quiet and
the surrounding streets provided
serious airs of higher seeing
that often led to a larger life
that was key to a Beat Generation
and the Beat refusal
to stand by much of anything
that led to smug conformity.

But funk and quiet rooms
didn't always lead to a larger life
but to a need to go out—
out on any road to somewhere—anywhere
where questions demanded experience
before they were answered.

To me, the Village then
was a place where all kinds
of free minded others
circled the old and the new critics
and rare friends who knew
when and where to ask
what time it was
in order to stop or nod
as if there was always time
to sip another espresso
before noticing a lonely loner
who seemed to know
what was needed by anyone—anywhere
was to simply see that
whatever was happening it was necessary
to know what to do
with the Beat of Beat poetry
which dealt with
how and why things were done.

Yet, in Greenwich Village in 2013
little seems to have changed
Café Reggio still serves espresso
and the tables and chairs are seldom empty.

Walking the streets of the Village
I'm reminded of my own time
when I turned eighty-three
when I forget things
I might have to remember
and remember things
I should forget.
Still, I am reminded that time is
no longer immaterial to
any place in America
because in 2013
America is still
haunted by the longest war
in its history
while more homes are disturbed
and more and more Americans
live in anxious fear of losing jobs.

In present economic straits
of political deceit
there is a growing sense of betrayal
and anger with blame
because America is gutted
by corporate greed
and political side games
eliminating the ground of middle class America
and splitting the fabric of our country
with a long black shadow
of some corporate MOLOCH!
The MOLOCH that

Allen Ginsberg "Howled" at
back in the 1950s
and who now is revisiting us
in our present time.

A Moloch that not only thrives
in climates of confusion and separation
but of men and women brain-washed
by lies and deceit
of self-serving pundits and politicians
who lack compassion
or realize that the growing needs of
the poor and hungry
are not caused by a lack of will to work
but the lack of work itself.

The kind of faith that makes America great
comes from a belief in change
and purpose that reveals wider horizons of
    opportunity
and chances to expand the conviction
of what we can do
versus what we cannot do
this inspires a focus
on what is possible right now.

For everything occurs in Now
the Now of present time
as T.S. Eliot reminds us
All time is eternally present
all time is unredeemable

what might have been
point to one end,
which is always present. . . .

So, my return to Greenwich Village
returns me
to the timelessness of Now
where I can always choose to believe
decline and separation
or return
to what our America was founded on:
the pursuit of happiness,
freedom
and justice for all
is possible
if we act in the Now
and remember
that in the power of freedom
and dissent
all is possible—
anything is possible.

R.B.

DIANA

Life in New York wasn't what we had expected. Robert's sister died in New Jersey shortly after we arrived. Fortunately, they were able to connect before she passed away. Robert saw his nephew and nieces at his sister's memorial; it was the last time he got to see them.

His daughter and son-in-law's new business made it difficult for them to spend time with us. I connected with a Zen group in White Plains and once a week took Robert to join them in meditation.

He enjoyed sitting with them in quiet contemplation and he hardly complained except when it was winter and their meditation space was cold and drafty. But Robert always felt cold in New York, especially when the temperature dropped below the 60s; he stayed bundled in layers, struggling in his "human condition," wearing long underwear beneath his Levi's or corduroy pants, a long sleeve undershirt beneath a regular shirt, and a sweater or cardigan, until summer.

And, the days when we weren't off to Manhattan, we'd walk in the neighborhood to a small park nearby. He'd sit on a bench and wait for me as I took a fast walk around several blocks ahead and back. It was a way to clear my head and troubled heart as much as exercise. During that time, he never gave me any cause for worry that he'd wander away and get lost. I'd say, "Be right back," and he'd smile and wave me away. He'd watch birds or squirrels or children play, or even better, an airplane crossing the sky overhead—something that so appealed to him, it made me wonder if it represented his lost freedom, physically or mentally.

34

A Human Condition

DIANA

A HUMAN CONDITION

How sensitive he's become
to the tone of my voice,
or any voice that speaks to him.
A tone, please, to set the pace
for lightness and ease.
He's forgetting how to wear clothes—
the order of things,
needs prompting:
simple clothes
laid out in the morning.
It's cold in New York's winter
so layering is the norm
but not easy—
clothes on the bed
now seem all the same to him.
Long underwear first, he's told:
examining the front and back

a balancing act
of one foot in,
then the other
careful not to fall.
The undershirt with its long sleeves,
then a turtleneck—how do
the hands go through
and over the neck—
he needs help
pulling it down the back.
The buttons, o, the buttons
one at a time for shirts
hands shake, pulling them through
how difficult it all is.
Hard to bend at eighty-five
to put socks on next.
To bring each over toes and up
before negotiating pants—
one leg in at a time
it helps to sit down.
Now slippers—or shoes
For indoor or out.
All the things
once done without thought
a puzzle as each day passes.

D.S.

Even though he couldn't remember the name of our
street or the number of our house, still, if he had to lead the
way, he'd more or less find it. I always checked his Medic

Alert bracelet that he faithfully wore for me. The best walks we took were at Glen Island Park on the Long Island Sound, where he loved to see the geese and ducks, the white, majestic swans, the cormorants perched on pilings, gulls diving in the water or landing near park benches for scraps of food. And always, he'd stop and gaze at airplanes, flying into "that blue sky" that, for Robert, seemed "bluer" wherever he was.

I once asked him what he felt about his life. It was a random question, hoping to probe into whatever was in his mind at the time. Robert answered, "My father used to say life is good, but you have to pay for it sometimes. When you do, it can get better but it can never be just right."

When he turned and asked me what people now thought of him when they came to see him, I'd say, "People come because they love you for what you are. They know you may not understand or always be able to respond, yet when you do, it's usually meaningful, if not humorous."

Sometimes we'd have care-persons come and be with him as I took off on appointments or errands. He never minded; he always encouraged me to go "see a friend," or take a tea lesson with a Japanese teacher I met when we arrived in New York. Yet I couldn't know what he was truly thinking or what was daily being processed through his fading memory. How is it, I thought, that after three decades and more, the mystery of him is still present? Words are said, understood, but I ask myself, do I truly listen? Or do I just listen to the words spoken in my own mind while processing his? Sometimes the love I feel is so acute I wonder how I might slip into his skin and head and ease his loss. How possible is it to slip into someone else's skin? To be that particular heart beat? It can only be possible when there's no experience of separation. Caring, isn't difficult—there just didn't seem enough of it at times.

John Zeisel, in his book *I'm Still Here*, points out the importance of the almond-shaped organ in the brain called the amygdala that processes our emotions, "particularly the emotions of anger and hate—but also love and caring" and how the amygdala stays "healthy far into the disease making people with Alzheimer's exquisitely sensitive to emotional events and other people's emotional states." (*I'm Still Here* p. 77–78.)

How true. We never lost the ability to communicate emotionally in a loving way far into Robert's disease.

And it is also true that the creative process in the brain, however limited by Alzheimer's, remains accessible. The sensitivity to sound, to visual or verbal arts, endures. The enjoyment of music, whether classical or jazz, country music or pop; sharing of a poem; a trip to the museum—these were all activities that not only brought joy but continual engagement with life in a meaningful and dignified way.

We were ever grateful to the Museum of Modern Art. The Meet Me At MOMA series was an interactive discussion of specific Museum paintings for participants with dementia accompanied by members of their family or caregivers. These meaningful monthly meetings were facilitated by specially trained Museum instructors. At one of the "Meet Me At MOMA" events, it was wonderful to see the entire exhibition of Paul Gauguin, for example, to view up close not only his paintings but wood carvings, and understand the strength of his designs and his use of warm, rich colors.

"Like that one," Robert said as he stood in front of one of Gauguin's nudes, *Tahitian Eve*. I remember reading, in his memoir, that Gauguin conceived life "as an existential struggle to reconcile."

Taking in Gauguin's art as he did, Robert mentioned "as great a painter as Gauguin was, how he must have suffered to create such work." From what depths did that come from? It was not Alzheimer's talking—or was it?

Later, I wondered why, when a research of the "Meet Me At MOMA" program found significant improvements in the temperaments of Alzheimer's patients and their care-persons, such art programs weren't being adopted in all dementia centers and museums nationally. Such a simple yet effective way to lift, honor, and dignify anyone with dementia. I was grateful to ARTZ in Massachusetts for initiating such a program and attempting to interest museums in other states in similar programs. Creating more engagement in the arts and music, whether in museums or theaters, or even in aging facilities, encouraging writing and poetry besides exercise, offers an alternative perspective to aging.

Robert brought his own view about aging.

35

Aging

ROBERT, 2012, NEW YORK

At eighty-three, barring memory loss, I seem to be unusually fit, which I attribute to genes and careful eating and physical exercise, which includes regular long walks.

Often, in a group of elderly people, some moan about aging and physical problems—complaints that become boring. When I mention eighty-three, I think, maybe I am too old for some and too young for others—yet I really can't care. Calling myself "elderly" locks me out of what I want to do and be.

In conversation with elders, I seldom mention age. For me it's a needless point as age should not necessarily be discussed since it differs among people. Aging involves luck as well as a person's ability to take care of the mind as well as the body. For me, another way of coping with aging that has helped me in numerous ways is a practice of Zen meditation.

As my wife Diana reminds me, "Age has little to do with aging. It is the quality of energy experienced moment by moment."

36

Existential Aging

ROBERT, 2013, NEW YORK

So, approaching eighty-four, brings me to a realization that—instead of measuring life in months and years—there is another view, which is to see life as nature does in seasons and change.

It can be said that perhaps I am in the last season of my life. Yet if this is so—there is a spring coming to bring a fresh beginning.

Life in a larger sense of the word never ends—it only changes where a whole new world arises.

So I am still a free human being, one person who loves what he lives and lives what he loves, never minding the rights and wrongs that seem to circle the hopes of everyone— the young as well as the old, the honest as well as others who seldom experience their own lives, often living without realizing what they can and cannot do in America, where change can always be had by those who know when to change, and what to change for their own good and the good of others.

After eighty-three years, I am aware and feel fine about all that I have done for others and all they have done for me.

This seems like a life of wonderful changes and of wonderful people who still seek what is new, and what is known—and—what will lead into the unknown. Life honest and seriously shared.

Yet as every day and week goes by and I grow older, I cannot help but wonder when my end will come; when that great "distinguished thing" will visit and take me away. This is something God alone knows, and I graciously leave it to Him because He seems to still keep me here for a reason!

However, in my present circumstance, I find I am able to experience more life, joy and wonder just by seeing those I know and love—and occasionally enjoying a Pale Ale too!

* * *

Sometimes just receiving a loving, friendly phone call from a friend makes me feel vital and joyful. I enjoy the fact that someone thought of me during his or her day or night.

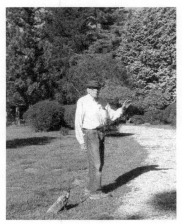

I still have that Beat need to go—go on by—just by living more life and at some point coming to my own end, whenever that might be. We won't entirely understand the various paths in our lives, and the reasons for them, until we are on the "other side."

Robert, Hammond Museum Garden, North Salem, NY, 2012.
Photo by Diana Saltoon

37
Friends

DIANA

FRIENDS

Temporary
clouds cross a sky
bigger than a world
of changes.
Time and circumstance
set us apart—
But like the sky unhindered—
friendship endures.

                              D.S.

The winter of 2014 in New York was brutal with a series
of relentless snowstorms. Ice and snow confined us indoors,
and even with the heat turned up in the house, we could
never feel warm enough. We mostly stayed indoors in the
fear we'd slip and fall on icy paths outside.

I made a radical decision—a road trip to Florida to
sunshine and warmth! We'd visit friends we hadn't seen

in years and carefully map out our route so I'd only drive during the day when it was still light and when the weather was clear.

It was kind of a last on-the-road trip for Robert, one last Beat experience. His daughter wondered at the sagacity of such a venture that would expose him to unfamiliar surroundings and even more confusion. Although her Alzheimer's concerns were valid and I did share them somewhat, I never doubted Robert's sense of curiosity and exploration and felt that as long as I could keep him safe and comfortable, we could slowly venture on and trust in the flow of our trip.

"Buckle up, Briggs," I'd say. "Adventure time!" as we got into the Camry and Robert duly buckled up. It was something I often said whenever we'd get into the car for a trip to New York City to visit friends or braved a longer trip to Becket, to the country home of some lifelong friends. Life always seemed one long adventure to me. Robert felt the same even about death.

So, we went to Florida. Our destination: Delray Beach, where a relative, who had generously invited us to stay, lived.

Along the way we connected with loving friends, former publishing colleagues and writers, and friends in Virginia and North Carolina who were thrilled to be reunited with Robert after many years, even as they found him different and faltering in words.

In Florida, we experienced a luxurious haven in which we relaxed under sunny skies. Our hospitable relative never minded when Robert lost his way, wandering into her private wing of the house as he searched for our bedroom.

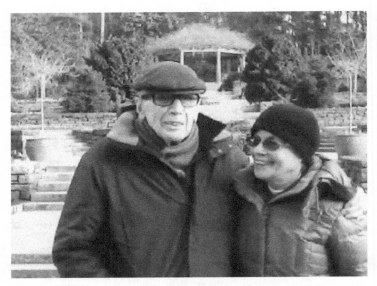

Robert and Diana, on-the-road trip from New York to Florida, 2014. (Photo taken by a passerby on Diana's camera.)

All during the trip, whether luck or intuition followed us, we managed to miss one February storm after another that hit the East Coast from Maine to North Carolina. All the roads we traveled were clear of snow and ice until, reaching our hometown again, we found our neighborhood still slick with patches of ice and curbs piled high with snow.

Our Florida road venture was an experiment that turned out to be the best escape from an otherwise inescapable winter. Rather than focus on the negative aspects of Alzheimer's disease and its debilitating future, I focused on Robert, his life as experienced moment-to-moment, and his responses. I found his acceptance and curiosity humanly noble and inspiring. They handed me a way to live more vividly as—like it or not—he continually drew me to the present, into the larger awareness and acceptance of life—*just as it is*—with all of its sharp edges. Being present in awareness increased the compassionate relationship we shared, which included all others and nature itself.

I believed the road trip, as crazy as it must have seemed to others, lifted and empowered Robert.

ROBERT, 2014, NEW YORK

Oh!!
Far away and
back again!
Friends we
should
never have
left
behind!
They were so
kind.
So kind.

R.B.

DIANA

Robert wrote that poem as we made plans to leave New York and return to Portland. It wasn't just the winter weather that helped us make this decision. We missed our circle of friends in Portland, friends who were more of an extended family. We missed Portland itself, a city that offered a slower pace than what we were experiencing in New York, although leaving his daughter was difficult. Robert's own primary care doctor felt he would benefit from a more "peaceful environment" and did not think the move would be detrimental to his condition.

We left New York when spring turned to summer.

38

"Shall We Dance?"

DIANA

It is dinnertime in our apartment in Portland, Oregon, August of 2014. The air is mild, the evening still light with the sun shimmering on leaves of dogwood trees outside our living room window, casting their shadows on an adjacent white wall in the room.

We're having mahi-mahi burgers with onions sautéed in coconut oil and a green salad we both share, some sweet potato chips on the side. Robert's enjoying an India Pale Ale while I nurse a glass of white wine as we listen to Nat King Cole on an old CD singing "Fascination."

Robert's head moves in appreciation of music and song and, all of a sudden, he reaches for his glass and pours some of his beer in my wine glass. "Toast!" he says, unaware he's mixed his beer with my white wine. I lift my glass and smile and we toast "to life together."

Then, amazingly, he gets up, says: "Dance?" Surprised, I say "yes" and we sway a bit to Cole's "Fascination." I say, "In Hawaii they clapped after we danced."

(That was so long ago, I thought to myself, a kind of late honeymoon in 1978 after our marriage in San Francisco a year earlier. We were at the Maui Intercontinental Hotel dining in their fancy dining room above the Maui shores. And we did dance! To live music of that time, to a tune I cannot recollect except it was more than a two-step dance, something like a combination of jazz and swing where he turned and dipped me almost to the ground as a grand finale.)

With Cole singing the old song, it is barely a two-step dance in our humble Portland apartment. Swaying to the music, hardly moving, he says, "They clap all over the world when you dance with me."

We sit back down to resume our meal. His goes half eaten but he continues to enjoy his beer. My wine is quite undrinkable and discretely I empty the glass in the sink; pour myself another before joining him again.

Where once he adored food and would never waste any, more and more, he is leaving food on his plate uneaten, food I reluctantly throw away or save for another meal at another time.

Robert's confusion of beer and wine is only another indication of the deepening progress of his dementia.

We are in the "independent living" building of a larger complex that includes an assisted living center as well as an Alzheimer's care facility.

Ours is a two-bedroom apartment, large enough for our needs. True, it is smaller than any place we had ever lived in, but we find it comfortable, full of light, and its surroundings well landscaped. More important, there is an air of tranquility about the place. There is a courtyard where we can quietly sit and watch the sun set late on a summer's day.

39

Remembering

DIANA

REMEMBERING

He moans at night
"Oh God, Oh God,"
is it some chronic pain.
Or is he bemoaning
something's wrong
and not knowing what to do
about its haunting.
Or is it some regret
that comes and goes
and stirs unbidden emotions.
Yet his energy is alive
and still strong
even in a body
grown thin in arms and legs
no fat to temper
a growing frailty.

At eighty-five he refuses a cane.
Why need one
when he still has me
to lend a shoulder or hand.

Love abounds
and we go on
this mystery way of Alzheimer's
I say to him,
"let me remember for you."

D.S.

The summer of 2014 is a sweet summer, warm, mild, breezy, with hardly any rainy days. There are many afternoon teas when friends come and visit and patiently hear Robert reading from something he'd written in New York. Some of them become care-persons for him, providing me with respite and allowing me to keep appointments and errands without Robert's presence. He experiences more difficulty waking up in the mornings and starting his day because his nights are frequently interrupted by pain in his chest and ribs, or the need to use the bathroom.

Writing is still something he never gives up. We have to have an exercise, I tell him. Try writing the alphabet from A to Z so you recognize them. He recites the letters almost perfectly, though misses some. The struggle to write and his determination to do so is heroic and, in spite of the frustration he feels, he accepts it and doesn't complain.

He no longer keeps time. The clock and its hands are a puzzle though he tries to draw the circle of time with its two hands. Time is of no consequence to him anyway. It is just the moment that counts.

He uses "white-out" fluid to edit or a pencil to add what words he can remember on a page. Surrounding himself with books, he picks one and leafs through it. It is the book he's written—*Ruined Time*—his 1950s memoir, and it helps jolt memories of his life. Somehow just handling books brings him comfort, an engagement in the literary world he loves.

Poetry always stimulates him, even the handling of pages of old poems he'd written. It brings him great pleasure whenever friends visit and encourage him to read a poem aloud. He especially enjoys reading his poem: *Time & San Francisco*. When reading that particular poem, it is as if some part of him returns and his attention to the words on the page comes alive, and his reading reflects a resonance reminiscent of "old Briggs." Friends are amazed and delighted to experience his voice and passion again, and, in spite of his affliction, he is still the consummate poet. For a while he is able to burst out of his bubble of forgetfulness, only to return to the bubble when setting the pages down again.

His love of jazz is ever present. Whenever a friend contacts us about a jazz group or gig, we try to join them. We reconnect with members of his Portland jazz trio and, whenever possible, attend their events. "How he must miss doing his reads to jazz," someone says, though I never hear a complaint, just the joy on his face when he hears live, cool jazz. "Happy?" I ask. He nods. I say, "I wish I could make others happy too." He pauses and says, "It's impossible to make anyone happy. Only they can make themselves happy. So all you can do is point out to them that they have to make themselves happy. That's how you help."

We take daily walks and join a weekly "gentle yoga" class on chairs. And there is meditation with a group of friends who never fail to welcome Robert, help him to a chair for meditation. Joining them requires him to be up earlier. As difficult as all these ventures are, he humors me and bravely attempts the activities even as it becomes more difficult to maneuver in and out of our small used car. Refusing a cane or walker—or God forbid—"the wheelchair," an obliging arm or hand is all Robert needs to keep on walking and moving.

He forgets many things but always remembers his favorite hat that has become his signature, a traditional Irish brown tweed wool cap.

Music continues to be an intrinsic part of our daily lives: in the morning, a favorite meditative CD; later, Chopin or the classical music channel. At night there is the jazz of Bill Evans or a local musician, or a CD of Billie Holiday. Once, listening to the haunting strains of *Romance of the Gadfly*, we reflect on better times back in the 1990s when we'd listen for hours to that same music.

Happiness is seeing Robert eat heartily. Where once this was a normal affair, now he just looks at the plate in front of him and lets the food go cold. His appetite has shrunk and his taste buds seem to have deserted him. I try serving more finger foods so he doesn't have to struggle with cutlery. Some of his favorites: coconut shrimp, egg rolls, tortilla chips with salsa, pizza, bread and cheese, and, best of all, a grilled cheese sandwich. He likes his bottle of beer—a Pale Ale that he pours in a glass I give him.

He no longer eats salads, greens of any kinds, vegetables or rice. Even his nutrition drink doesn't cut it anymore with him, although he takes a few sips at night now and then. Perhaps he doesn't remember how or why to eat and not eat.

40

Opus "22"

DIANA

OPUS "22"

An afternoon in SE Portland
soft rain falling
its rhythm on the window
in tune to Chopin's 22.
He turns to the music
head tilting, joy on his face
as he keeps pace
with the tempo
of rain and piano.

I hold his latest words
on a sumie pad someone gave

"What do I do
    when
    I only have
    you
    to call on?

When you have
gone away
and, no longer here?
Even though
you assure me
you will never
leave . . ."

The writing continues in his head
even though words are lost—
they come and go
and when they stay
they appear on the pad
then disappear,
disappear.

D.S.

As summer turns to fall and winter approaches, it is evident that Robert is slipping into a deeper stage of his disease.

Washing dishes after dinner. As I face the sink, I'm suddenly overwhelmed with sadness and tears fall unchecked as I go on washing dishes. It is something I try not to give in to. Robert is in the bedroom. He has taken his shoes off, put on his slippers and lies on the bed with his clothes on. A sob escapes and I try to hide the fact that I'm crying but can't stop myself. It's hard loving someone so much that it hurts.

Then, I feel his arms around me. Somehow he sensed my tears. He moves me around toward his chest and hugs me. "I will always be with you," he says. "Everywhere." Then he makes two fists with his hands and tells me to do the same. "Spread your arms wide," he says. I follow what he wants me to do. With our hands in fists and arms wide, he looks at me, smiles and opens his hands. "There, just let go," he says. "I loved you the day I saw you, that first time we met in San Francisco."

This isn't Alzheimer's talking, this is Robert. He knows—he's cognizant, and he wants me to know how loved I am and how he will go on loving me no matter what. This makes me cry even more, although I know he mustn't see me cry or know I'm sad. There will be repercussions from this outburst of mine, but now I just feel the warmth of him holding me and leading me to rest on the bed. "Come, come and lay with me. Look at me." We stay, holding each other and looking at each other. Instead of me comforting him, he comforts me.

This is Robert, always seeing how he can give, how he can make things easier for me. He tells me he needs to turn within himself more. "Meditate." Not to go anywhere particularly to do this, "just here." While lying in bed, this is what he tries to do. "It is," he says, "more important now."

41

Portland, 2015

DIANA

New Year's Eve came uneventfully. Robert went to bed early as I sat meditating the minutes through the turn of the year. Fireworks in the distance told me the hour of midnight had come, and 2015.

The fireworks woke him up and he joined me in the living room. We toasted in the New Year with a small cup of sake I had poured for us. We sat across the table as I served soba noodles—a symbol of longevity. His bowl of noodles went untouched, but he finished off his sake, saying he wasn't hungry.

2015 found Robert still in fairly good spirits, joining in activities I planned. He valiantly went with another companion, a younger man, more like a son to him, on excursions to a garden, acupuncture sessions, a yoga class, or to a restaurant for pizza or a grilled cheese sandwich he shared, leaving his half-eaten.

Subtly, but surely, his condition took a further dip in the following weeks and months as he completely lost appetite and ate and drank less. Even his nutritional drinks, always handy in the refrigerator, were hardly touched. I saw him steadily lose more weight and worried about possible dehydration.

What was really going on? Once, bending down to fasten his shoes, I felt his hand on my head. Looking up, I saw him shake his head. I looked at him with a question on my lips I knew he wouldn't—or couldn't answer. "How is it really with you?"

He just shook his head and said, "No more." With hands on my shoulders, he tried to help me up.

It was early May. On a checkup with his doctor, I was alarmed when she took me aside and suggested "Hospice"—even as she told me his vitals were normal. Robert heard the "H" word and was silent.

As shocked as I was at the doctor's suggestion, I faced the inevitable and made an appointment the following week with a hospice nurse and social worker. Two days before the appointment, Robert complained of acute pain in his lower chest and abdominal area that kept him up all night even with the help of his usual over-the-counter pain medication. The next morning a friend came and we took Robert to the VA emergency room where he waited for hours in a wheelchair. I gave him more pain medication which seemed to help. He hardly complained the entire time except for being cold. It was warm outside but he felt the air condition vent close by his wheelchair. There was no place comfortable to move him in the room filled with waiting patients. A nurse handed him a warm blanket but it was obvious he was in a great deal of discomfort.

Later we found out his pain was due to pancreatitis and the inability to empty his bladder.

He spent the night at the VA hospital in a room of his own with a great view of Portland, but he was hardly aware of it. Tired out from the previous night with no sleep, now sedated and finally without pain, he slept soundly.

The ER doctor advised me to contact Robert's daughter in New York. She was already planning to be in Portland in two weeks, but the doctor felt she should come sooner. And so I called her, and still in distress, returned home to an empty apartment where it struck me—oh, so sharply, so glaringly, that I was losing Robert.

42

Departure

DIANA

DEPARTURE

Our home an open door
welcomed friends
coming and going,
gifts of love,
food and flowers
sustained us with their solace.
A guest came in unseen
and quietly took you away.
Done with debilitation and
confusion—how ready you were.
You took a last breath
then, no more.
That last guest
who took you gently
left behind a precious gem—
the best of all inheritance—
your love that never dies.

D.S.

Hospice was but a short time. Four days to be exact. Robert passed peacefully just thirteen days before his eighty-sixth birthday. Much can be said about a man who loved and lived with dignity, grace, and kindness. Gifted and creative to his end, Robert entered death with a light heart and loving soul. He was surrounded by his family of close friends and by Hillary, his daughter, his "kid."

Much later, while leafing through his papers, I found a discarded envelope where he tried to scribble a message to me, two weeks before he died.

And yes, as in most times, he did get the last word in.

> Oh!
> oh! no—
> wife!
> Just let!!! Go
> R . B .

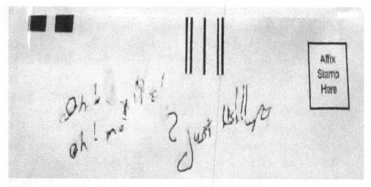

Discarded envelope with Robert's last words barely discernible.

Epilogue

The greatest thing in a man
is not what he's accomplished but how he loved.

R.B.

DIANA

In a guest book Hillary began when her Dad was in hospice, I look over what I wrote the week after he passed to make some sense of my life now without him:

Robert died on Friday, May 29, 2015. He didn't wait for the month's end, or his next birthday on June 11 when he'd turn eighty-six. Perhaps he didn't want to be eighty-six. A few days before his death, Robert thought of his dad who died at eighty-two, his sister, his mother. His dad, dying at eighty-two—or was it eighty-three? "How old am I now?" he'd ask, as I held his hand a week before he went. "Still a kid," I'd say. "No, I think I'm eighty-three."

What did it ever matter about his age? So many comments about him at his memorial, thoughts of others, I'll get them all together somehow, I said to myself. There was jazz at his memorial. Some members of his trio came. How Robert must have loved them turning out for him. Tim on drums, Andre on bass, young Ian on sax. And all his Portland friends who came to say something about him, an entertainer from New York, and Mark, a dear, trusted friend from San Francisco—and yes, your own "kid," Hillary, "were there in full force," I said aloud. It was a great celebration of your life with music, poetry and stories, with tears, laughter, and joyful remembrances.

We buried a third of your ashes in the Veterans Cemetery in SE Portland. That too, was quite a moving tribute. They placed a stone later over your ashes with the words: "The Beat Goes On." Can't remember who actually thought that one out—Hillary, I think. She took a third of your ashes with her, leaving me the rest of you, most of which I scattered in the Pacific. There are still some ashes left. I can't seem to let this last bit of you go just yet, even though you remind me not to cling—to "let go."

Grief has become a part of my being. Unfamiliar with this companion, I'm at sea, unsure how to steer my new life as it is, especially when my mind narrows down to emotions and there's just pain. Thoughts rush in. Why didn't I hold him more? So many *whys,* so many *chides.* How I could have done better for him? During the last year, so immediate seemed each moment-to-moment intensity—of waking him, showering him, dressing him, doing those buttons and shoes, then trying to coax him into eating a breakfast: all of these activities robbed me of awareness of his actual presence. Yet I would do those activities wholeheartedly again, just for the pleasure of touching him, still alive, still present. Thirty-eight years together! Such a gift of himself in every way to his very end. He despaired of not "making it" materially for Hillary and me. No one could know how hard he worked. How he wrote daily from morning to night, those reads he loved to do with his jazz trio. How much he appreciated them. How he loved jazz. When we returned to Portland, he enjoyed the music I'd play for him each day. His head moving side to side with the music, feeling each beat beating into his heart, giving it his whole attention. So present, so alive, harmoniously blending in each moment.

I join a grief counseling group but find little relief. Each experience is unique to each person. How can one make a chart of grief or find a ready solution? In the mail I finally receive something I can resonate with. It's from a Hospice Bereavement Program provided by the hospice company that helped with Robert's care. In the newsletter is an article by Alan D. Wolfelt, Ph.D., Director of the Center for Loss & Life Transition, in Ft. Collins, Colorado. He writes of five common myths regarding grief: that grief and mourning are the same experience; that there is a predictable and orderly progression of grief; that one moves away from grief and mourning instead of toward it; that tears expressing grief are only a sign of weakness; and, that the goal is to get over one's grief.

I find his explanations helpful. Mourning is different from grief, a way to outwardly express inner thoughts and emotions when we lose our loved one. No one likes to see someone cry. We "shush" a baby when it cries, so a grown-up too, is encouraged, in a way, to stop crying. Embarrassment, too, is an issue. I hardly ever break down in front of friends, no matter how loving they are, to "spare" them. But now I understand it's more healing to do so, to give into tearful outbreaks, especially when a strong, loving shoulder of a dear friend is offered.

We so want to make sense of our grief—we even think of stages in grief. How simple if all grief could be neatly categorized in boxes and discarded at some stage. But, since my grief is different from another's, how can anyone say when it will ever end?

I think of that last myth that Dr. Wolfelt mentions: "getting over" grief and returning to normalcy. What is normal for me now? Robert's death has forever changed me. The desolate depth of my loss is acutely present, but grief shows a way to see life differently, more clearly. Impermanence is no longer an intellectual understanding. Intensely experienced up-close and real, it points to the reality in which the dream world of impermanence assures us that all experiences *pass*—that the recurring waves of grief are what they are—waves that come and go and change and yes, that even this sadness I feel is a dream. Hard to accept, in my human form of rising emotions.

I continue the music at home, although the music without Robert brings sweet sadness for his missing heartbeat. The nights are particularly hard. I cross my arms around my chest and rock back and forth crying aloud. Sometimes I don't know if I can go on without him. Don't know how or why. I no longer want to live. I'd rather die. I want to join him in death. And, as I cry, a voice in my ear says, "I didn't release you for this." I feel his presence reminding me I'm not alone; I remember his words, "I shall always be with you, I'll always love you." My heart calms and breathing deeply, I find peace.

A week will go by until something small, unforeseen, triggers grief—a note I left for him that falls out of a book saying, "Robert, I'll be right back," or hear the same tune played when we last had a meal together, or a photograph. The emotional head of grief rears and wipes away the peace, leaving me again in pain. The *now* brings this up too. A surge of sadness unexpectedly floods a vulnerable heart.

Sogyal Rinpoche's *The Tibetan Book of Living and Dying*, gives a positive aspect to my grief besides the truth of impermanence. It teaches me to accept loss and anguish and meet them in the heart with loving compassion. There is an essence of shining clarity, a home beyond birth and death, beyond all emotions, beyond this living world of dreams where all things arise and pass, an all-embracing essence where Robert has returned.

I am reminded to meditate more. There is no separating from the essence that holds us all as we dance together in it. And here, I realize with joy, Robert and I meet as one again. Grief brings me here, now, to this realization.

"You are forever teaching me," I say to him. "Even now you teach me how to handle this sorrow. Teaching me that every time I forget and separate from our essence the tears come. Staying in our essence, in the awareness of now, my heart returns home to peace and oneness with you." So simply true, so simply real.

I shall probably forget then remember again, though I expect that my new companion, this grief that has become a living part of me, will return my heart home again, and again to you.

> The moon wakens me from a dream.
> Bright and transparent,
> its light floods in.
> And, out there in the sky,
> free, like the star's sparkle,
> unhindered, unbounded, you smile,
> lifting the darkness from my soul.
>
> D.S.

Acknowledgments

DIANA

Making this book a reality was possible because of many friends, colleagues, and family members who lent a hand along the way and generously contributed to the early funding of the project. My thanks to all of you including my brother, Elias Saltoon, his wife Lilian, Stephen Friedland, Carolyn Winkler, Moira Bell, Linda Nelson, Angie Gasq, Myrna Begin, Floyd Ottoson, Jan Waldmann, Joanna and Bob Meyer, Tracy Koslicki, Carl Viggiani, Patricia Reid, Audrey Larsen, James Bates, and Christopher Hodgson.

To Jane Wilcox and Anita Jones for your early editorial assistance and advice and to photographer, Mark Eifert.

Special thanks to Noah Devros, Christine Toth, and Steve Arndt, for your hands-on help with the project throughout its inception and for your unfailing encouragement and support. To Mark Ong of Side By Side Studios for your kindness, generosity, advice, and above all, taking on the design of the book, and to Susan Riley, his assistant. To Peyton Stafford for your compassion, understanding, and continual help and concern, to editor Suzanne Copenhagen, and to Merloyd Lawrence and Laura Stanfill, for help with publishing suggestions.

To Hillary Sheperd, who guided her father and me in New York, as we began our Alzheimer's journey. Her research and assistance were invaluable, as were the Alzheimer's Association, all of the literature and books that opened a wealth of information on the disease, including Joanne Koenig's book *Leaning to Speak Alzheimer's* and John Zeisel's book, *I'm Still Here*, that provided key information, encouragement, and inspiration, and to Sean Caulfield, co-founder of ARTZ (Artists for Alzheimer's).

Gratitude to those who took care of Robert and me in many ways in New York and Portland, and to Deborah Green in Seattle. Countless thanks to Forrest Sheperd, Ann Vellis, Peter and Susan Matson, Russ Michael and his White Plains Zen Center sangha, and New York Zen teachers Daiken Nelson and Carl Viggiani, for your many kindnesses and understanding.

Profound appreciation to Sam Tyler and Bruce Rothman for accommodations between our moves from Portland and when we returned, to Chel and Laura White for anticipating our needs as we moved into our Portland apartment, your loyal friendship, concern, and encouragement never failed to lift us; thanks to Ruth Caplin, Patricia Reilly, Steve Lucia, Jean and J. D. Devros, Michelle Bagley, Ann Marsh, and Gary Fear; to Robert's jazz musicians and dear friends Stuart Fessant, Tim DuRoche, Andre St. James, and Dan Davis, for making Robert's reads possible, as well as sax player, Ian Christensen.

I'm most grateful to the sensitive care-persons who came willingly in New York and Portland to enable some time to myself, in particular Ted Bagley, who adopted us into his family and became a dear "son" to Robert during his last years and for still keeping an eye out for me; to Blythe Gatewood and Gina Quitorio for their loving patience especially in Robert's last weeks.

Gratitude to Moira Bell and Jill Romm for your compassion, counseling, and guidance when Robert was in hospice. Above all, deep appreciation to Jan Chozen Bays for aid in Robert's transition and continuing guidance with the process of grief; to Hogen Bays for his support; to Larry Christensen, Gyokuko Carlson, and members of the Zen communities in Oregon, Washington, and New York. Infinite gratitude to Shodo Harada Roshi and Priscilla (Chisan) Storandt for your ongoing Zen teachings, inspiration, and encouragement, and to the Chado tea community at large. The practices of Zen and Tea are profound pillars in my human journey of life and death.

Heartfelt thanks to others who have touched our lives in countless ways. Your sincere friendship, love, and understanding, enabled this book to come to its completion.

Bibliography

REFERENCES

Boyd, Doug. *Rolling Thunder*, New York: Random House, 1974. Published in Association with Robert Briggs Associates

Briggs, Robert. *Ruined Time: The 1950s and the Beat*. Portland, OR: Robert Briggs Associates, 2006

Coste, Joanne Koenig. *Learning to Speak Alzheimer's*. New York: Houghton Mifflin Company, 2003

Hanh, Thich Nhat. *The Miracle of Mindfulness*. Boston: Beacon Press, 1975.

Kornfield, Jack. *A Path with Heart: A Guide Through the Perils and Promises of Spiritual Life*. New York: Bantam Books, 1993

Miller, Henry. *The Air-Conditioned Nightmare*. New York: New Directions Publishing, 1945

Pelletier, Kenneth. *Mind as Healer, Mind as Slayer*. New York: Dell Publishing, 1977

Rinpoche, Sogyal. *The Tibetan Book of Living and Dying*. New York: HarperCollins, 1992

Schwartz, Jack. *The Path of Action*. New York: Plume – Penguin Books/Published in Association with Robert Briggs Associates, 1977.

Young, Arthur. *The Reflexive Universe*. New York: Delacourte Press/Merloyd Lawrence/Published in Association with Robert Briggs Associates, 1976. New Publication by Anados Foundation: Cambria, CA

————. *Which Way Out and Other Essays*, San Francisco: Robert Briggs Associates, 1980. New publication by Anados Foundation, Cambria, CA

Zeisel, John, PhD. *I'm Still Here*, New York: Penguin Group, 2010.

POETRY

Auden, W. H. *Collected Poems*. New York: Random House, 1976

Eliot, T.S. *The Wasteland, Prufrock and Other Poems*. New York: Dover Publications, Inc., 1998

Ginsberg, Alan. *Howl and Other Poems*. San Francisco: City Lights Books, 1956

Hardy, Thomas. *Selected Poems: Edited with an Introduction and Notes by Robert Mezey*. New York: Penguin Books, 1998

Jarrell, Randall. *Losses*. New York: Harcourt Brace, 1948

Olds, Sharon. *The Dead and the Living, Poems by Sharon Olds*. New York: Alfred A. Knopf, 1984

Patchen, Kenneth. *Selected Poems by Kenneth Patchen*. New York: New Directions, 1957

Poe, Edgar Allan. *The Complete Poetry of Edgar Allan Poe*. New York: Signet Classics, New American Library, a division of Penguin Group (USA) Inc., 1996.

Sandburg, Carl. *Smoke and Steel*. New York: Harcourt, Brace and Howe, Inc., 1920

Whitman, Walt. *Leaves of Grass*. New York: Dover Publications, Inc., 2007

SUGGESTED READINGS FOR CAREGIVERS

Brach, Tara, PhD. *Radical Acceptance*. New York: Bantam Books, 2003

Edson, Margaret. *Wit. A Play*. New York: Farrar, Straus and Giroux, 1999.

Eggleston, Georgena. *A New Mourning: Discovering the Gifts in Grief*. Bloomington, IN: Balboa Press, 2015

Kramer, Gregory. *Insight Dialogue*. Boston: Shambhala Publications, Inc., 2007

Shulman, Alix Kates. *To Love What Is*. New York: Farrar, Straus and Giroux, 2008

Tam, Jacqui. *A Daughter's Gift: Standing Tall*, Edmonton, Alberta: Iceberg Publishing, 2010

ZEN

Bancroft, Ann. *Zen, Direct Pointing to Reality*. London: Thames and Hudson, 1979

Bays, Jan Chozen Roshi. *How to Train a Wild Elephant & Other Adventures in Mindfulness*. Boston: Shambhala Publications, 2011

———. *Mindful Eating: A Guide to Rediscovering a Healthy and Joyful Relationship with Food*. Boston: Shambhala Publications, 2009

Harada, Shodo Roshi. *Morning Dewdrops of the Mind*. Berkeley: CA Frog, Ltd., 1993

———. *The Path to Bodhidharma*. Boston: Tuttle Publishing, 2000

Loori, John Daido. *The Zen of Creativity: Cultivating Your Artistic Life*. New York: Ballantine Books; Reprint edition, 2004

———. *The Art of Just Sitting*. Wisdom Publications: Somerville, MA, 2002

Thich Nhat Hanh. *Being Peace*. Berkeley, CA, Parallax Press, 1987.

———. *Fear: Essential Wisdom for Getting Through the Storm*. New York: HarperCollins Publishers, 2012

Watts, Alan. *The Way of Zen*. New York: Pantheon Books, 1957

———. *Beat Zen, Square Zen*. San Francisco: City Lights, 1959

Zuzuki, Shunryu. *Zen Mind, Beginner's Mind*. New York: John Weatherhill, Inc. 1970

THE BEAT GENERATION

Charters, Ann. *Kerouac, A Biography*. San Francisco: Straight Arrow Books, 1973

———, editor. *The Portable Reader*. New York: Viking Penguin Books, 1992

Ginsberg, Alan. *Howl and Other Poems*. San Francisco: City Lights Books, 1956

Kerouac, Jack. *On the Road, The Original Scroll*. New York: Penguin Group, 2007

Kyger, Joanne. *The Tapestry and the Web*. San Francisco: Four Seasons Foundation, 1965.

Meltzer, David. *Beat Thing*. Albuquerque, NM: La Alameda Press, 2004

———. *Tens, Selected Poems: 1961–1971*. New York: McGraw-Hill, 1973

THE WAY OF TEA

Hammitzsch, Horst. *Zen in the Art of the Tea Ceremony*. New York: St. Martin's Press, 1980

Okakura, Kakuzo. *The Book of Tea*. Rutland, VT and Tokyo, Japan: Charles E. Tuttle Co., Inc., 1956

Saltoon, Diana. *Tea and Ceremony: Experiencing Tranquility*. Portland, OR: Robert Briggs Associates, 2004

Sen, Shoshitsu XV. *The Enjoyment of Tea*. Japan: Tankosha, 2006

———. *The Spirit of Tea*. Japan: Tankosha, 2002

———. *Tea Life, Tea Mind*. New York: John Weatherhill, 1979.

Sen'o Tanaka. *The Tea Ceremony*. Tokyo, Kodansha International, 1973.

Yu, Lu. *The Classic of Tea*. Translated by Francis Ross Carpenter. Boston: Little, Brown and Co., 1974.

About the Authors

ROBERT BRIGGS

Robert Briggs attended Auburn and Columbia Universities and served in the U.S. Army during the Korean War. He became a partner in The San Francisco Book Company in 1972 and in 1973 founded Robert Briggs Associates, a group of West Coast consultants to writers and small publishers. The Association was involved in a variety of nonfiction publications including *Rolling Thunder* by Doug Boyd, *Mind as Healer, Mind as Slayer*, Kenneth R. Pelletier's classic book on stress, as well as works by Joseph Campbell, Stanislav Grof,

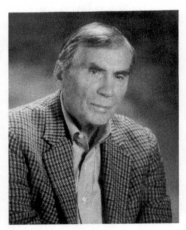

Robert, Portland, OR, 2001.
Photo by Mark Eifert

Colin Wilson, and Theodore Roszak. Briggs is also the author of *The American Emergency: A Search for Spiritual Renewal in an Age of Materialism*, 1986, and *Ruined Time: the 1950s and the Beat*, 2006. *Ruined Time* is a cultural autobiography of the Great Depression, World War II and the 1950s. This book sparked various multimedia projects including *Jazz and Poetry & Other Reasons*, reads written and read by Robert Briggs and accompanied by jazz musicians in performances in Portland, OR. CDs were produced that include *Poetry in the 1950s*

(1999), *Someone Said No* (2003), *My Own Atom Bomb* (2005), *The Beat Goes On* (2008), *Love in America* (2009), and *The Beat Revealed* (2011). Robert Briggs was involved in early West Coast jazz and poetry scenes where he performed in San Francisco's Jazz Cellar. To Briggs, "Jazz is to music, what poetry is to knowing."

DIANA SALTOON

Diana Saltoon has traveled extensively, studied yoga, and in the 1970s developed a program that dealt with modern stress. Her interest in Zen led to a study of Chado, The Way of Tea, as a Zen art and received a certificate of Chamei from the Urasenke School in Kyoto, Japan. Diana became a teacher at the Portland Wakai Tea Association in Oregon before moving with her husband, Robert Briggs, to New York in 2011. They returned to Portland, Oregon, in 2014.

A member of Zen communities in Oregon and New York, Diana continues to give presentations, classes, and workshops on the Zen Art of Tea. She is the author of *Tea and Ceremony: Experiencing Tranquility* (2004), *The Common Book of Consciousness* (1990), and *Four Hands: Green Gulch Poems* (1987).

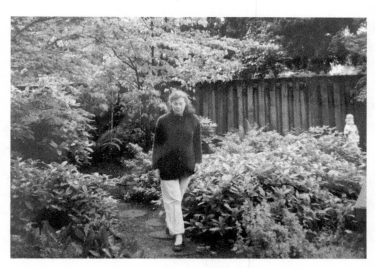

Diana on the garden path of their Oregon City home, OR, 1999.
Photo by Robert Briggs

CPSIA information can be obtained
at www.ICGtesting.com
Printed in the USA
BVHW04s0710010518
514725BV00001BA/33/P

9 780931 191206